Holistic Therapies

Helen McGuinness

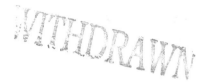
Hodder & Stoughton

A MEMBER OF THE HODDER HEADLINE GROUP

Orders: please contact Bookpoint Ltd, 39 Milton Park, Abingdon, Oxon OX14 4TD. Telephone: (44) 01235 400414, Fax: (44) 01235 400454. Lines are open from 9.00–6.00, Monday to Saturday, with a 24 hour message answering service. Email address: orders@bookpoint.co.uk

British Library Cataloguing in Publication Data
A catalogue record for this title is available from The British Library

ISBN 0 340 772964

First published 2000
Impression number   10 9 8 7 6 5 4 3 2
Year   2006 2005 2004 2003 2002 2001

Typeset by Wearset, Boldon, Tyne and Wear.
Printed in Great Britain for Hodder & Stoughton Educational, a division of Hodder Headline Plc, 338 Euston Road, London NW1 3BH by J.W. Arrowsmith Ltd., Bristol.

Contents

CHAPTER 6 — Aromatherapy

CHAPTER 7 — Reflexology

Acknowledgements

I would like to thank the following people for the help and support they have so kindly offered me whilst writing this book. Without their help this book would not have been turned into a reality.

Firstly to my husband Mark who continues to be a constant source of love, help, support and encouragement to me and has always believed in my abilities to write this book.

To my father Roy for his love and support and especially for his gift and skill in producing illustrations at such short notice, and to my mother Valerie for her love, encouragement and valued contributions, and especially for believing in me.

Dr Nathan Moss for so generously sharing his knowledge with me and especially for his considerable contributions, in particular to the Pathology and Stress Management chapters. Also for the hours he has taken out of his precious leisure time to read many of the chapters and offer his medical expertise and constructive comments.

To my special friends: Dee Chase who has constantly believed in my abilities, Sue Muir whose positive encouragement has been a source of inspiration to me and Annie Moss who has so generously offered her precious time to review the work and offer her valued contributions.

Thanks also go to Sue Muir and Sharon Holloway, who kindly offered their time to model for the photographs in this book, which were taken by Angus MacDonald.

Lastly thanks go to all the staff of the Holistic Training Centre who have made it possible for me to have the time to write this book and to all students who have supported and encouraged me to write.

Foreword

Complementary therapies are numerous. Some texts are written with a specific agenda to meet the needs of the individual therapist in their own speciality. Others are generally compiled with noticeable bias towards the author's interest and they go far beyond the needs of beginners, producing bulky texts which are restrictive in their context.

To find a book which combines comprehensive theory with practical skills in all aspects of complementary therapy is hard. To find all that together with an understandable, step-by-step guide to the benefits and application of various techniques, plus practical tips is a major bonus.

In writing such a book, Helen McGuinness has combined her extensive skills in most aspects of complementary therapy with her teaching and training abilities to produce a useful text for learners, beginners, therapists and trainers in any speciality of complementary therapy. It is also of interest to medical and nursing professionals who may find it a fascinating introduction to the type of therapies received by their patients. It will enable them to understand the rationale behind the use of complementary therapies and to appreciate their value, both within the setting of General Practice and in liaison with complementary practitioners.

Helen's pedigree in writing stems from her two highly successful books *Anatomy and Physiology – Beauty Therapy Basics* and *Aromatherapy – Therapy Basics*, along with the numerous training manuals and videos on aspects of complementary therapies.

Complementary therapists gain their skills and qualifications from a variety of schools, institutes and training centres. Their curriculum, modules and qualifying bodies are variable, with some common guidelines and validation. The rapid explosion of public interest in Complementary Therapy demands a safe delivery of this therapy with verifiable and accreditable training. The granting of the qualification should have measurable parameters to indicate that successful candidates have achieved the first step in their training to become safe and skilled therapists. The text is an essential guide for trainers and trainees to help them in their endeavour to maintain and improve their skills and practice in a professional manner.

I congratulate Helen on producing this book which will help to refresh those who are practising and will probably inspire the newcomers to aim for a recognisable and flourishing profession.

Dr Nathan Moss MBCh, B, MRCGP

Preface

Due to a substantial increase in the popularity of holistic health care, therapists are now looking to become multi-skilled in order to meet the demands placed on the growing industry of holistic therapies.

During my career to date as a beauty and holistic therapist, lecturer, assessor and verifier, I have seen a rapid rise in the popularity of holistic therapies, which are now gaining acceptance and credibility in many fields including the medical profession. Holistic therapists, therefore, need to be equipped with extensive knowledge and skills to help them deal with their clients successfully, and in order for them to be recognised as professionals in their own right.

This book is not designed to be a definitive guide to each therapy but aims to provide an essential and useful guide to practising holistic therapies to a safe and effective level.

It has also been written with the specific aims of addressing important issues such as client management, common pathological conditions, stress management, establishing a holistic therapy business, and to provide an introduction to more specialist subjects, such as understanding imbalance.

This book has been written primarily for holistic therapist students, qualified practitioners and trainers, but will also be of interest to nursing and medical professionals who wish to gain an understanding of the benefits and effects of holistic therapies and who may wish to pursue a career in this field.

Helen McGuinness

CHAPTER 1

History and development of holistic therapies

With the increase in the growth and development of holistic therapies in the 1990s and into the new millennium, it has become apparent that we are moving towards a profound structural change in our health care system.

The terms 'alternative' and 'unconventional' medicine have become outdated, as there has been a growing recognition of the value of holistic and complementary therapies in health care. With this, there is a greater need for therapists to become more professional and accountable for their individual therapies.

This chapter explores the concept of holistic therapies, and presents a perspective on how and why they have grown in popularity. More importantly, we look at how they can be used to subtly enhance more conventional methods of treating illness.

The term 'holistic therapies' is used loosely to describe a unique approach to treatment through a range of different therapies, rather than a medical concept or system.

Although the application of the word 'holistic' is relatively new, the concept of holistic health care goes back at least 2500 years to when Hippocrates, the father of holistic medicine, believed health was restored by facilitating a state of equilibrium within the fluid essences of the body. He stressed the importance of holistic therapies and placed great emphasis on proper diet and lifestyle. He used drugs to *support healing*, rather than to cure disease.

The opposing school of thought to Hippocrates held that a disease could be overcome with a specific cure. Later the scientific revolution of the nineteenth century brought with it the development of new drugs such as aspirin. The holistic concept of restoring balance and self-healing was abandoned in favour of drugs which appeared to have spectacular results by relieving symptoms.

The philosophical debate between conventional and complementary medicine is steeped in history. Conventional medicine defines ill health as specific identifiable symptoms, which are curable by specific treatments and/or drugs, whereas complementary medicine sees illness as an imbalance and disharmony within the body, with the physical symptoms as secondary manifestations. Conventional medicine defines health as being the absence of disease, as opposed to the holistic view which defines health as the complete state of physical, mental and social well-being.

During the first half of the nineteenth century the holistic concept of treatment was shunned and all but outlawed; some therapies were even branded as witchcraft! However, the 1990s in particular have witnessed a happy convergence of medical and complementary, or holistic, therapies towards what one may term 'medical pluralism'.

The unique feature of holistic or complementary therapies, despite the diversity of the individual therapies, is that they all aim to activate the self-healing capacity of the body and each has a theoretical base, linked by nature.

Holistic therapies differ from conventional medicine in that:
- Therapies work with symptoms and not against them. They aim to work with the normal functions of the body.
- The person's individuality is taken into account – each person's condition is different and, therefore, requires a different approach. In holistic health care no standard treatment can be appropriate for all individuals, or for individuals with the same condition.
- The treatment strategy aims to work towards physical and emotional well-being and not towards the absence of symptoms, as in conventional medicine. There is, therefore, no fixed beginning or end to the treatment, as the approach is one of preventative health care and maintenance of a state of well-being.
- The patient or client is an integral part of the process, with the emphasis on self-healing and the patient taking responsibility for their own health. The concept of holistic health care is not about an individual being the passive recipient of a cure.
- Holistic practitioners help clients to examine their lifestyle patterns as well as their bodily symptoms and work towards a long-term approach of restoring balance, rather than a short-term response to each incidence of disease.

The expansion in holistic and complementary therapies relates to the growing need to address the vast numbers of people suffering with stress-related illnesses, such as skin problems, digestive problems, heart disease and high blood pressure. There is a proliferation of media coverage of health-related problems as patients become more and more interested in how they can become an active part of restoring their physical and emotional well-being. Magazines and newspaper articles are full of testimonials from individuals who verify that holistic therapies, such as massage, aromatherapy and reflexology, have helped them with musculo-skeletal problems such as backache and arthritis, chronic pain as in headaches and migraines, allergies, cardiovascular problems, chronic immune-related problems such as ME, chronic infections like cystitis, and the non-specific conditions which are hard to diagnose by conventional medical techniques.

An increasing number of patients are now looking to holistic and complementary therapies for relief from failed medical treatment, due to a perceived lack of understanding of their condition or because they have experienced unpleasant side effects.

It would seem that, in the past, the principle school of thought in medicine has been blind to anything but disease. However, medicine is now starting to integrate some of the holistic concepts into health care, such as stressing the importance of changes in diet and lifestyle and reducing stress levels in cases of cardiovascular disease.

However, it should not be denied that in the process of accommodating both complementary and conventional medicine in our health care service, both systems will have areas of failure, as well as success. For instance, no amount of development in the field of complementary medicine could replace the excellence of traditional medicine in surgery, vaccinations and the control of acute infections.

Patients should receive traditional medicine for acute, life-threatening conditions in order to help sustain life. However, complementary forms of treatment, which may be used simultaneously with traditional treatment, can help patients to cope with their condition and effect the restoration of physical and emotional balance.

Complementary health practitioners are now starting to be acknowledged as professionals in their own right, as more and more doctors admit that, although they wish to learn more about complementary therapies, it is a diverse field which requires specific skills, knowledge and training.

It is interesting to note that the British Medical Association's educational requirement is for doctors to become sufficiently familiar with the forms of treatment available in complementary medicine to know what to expect from the related system and to decide who may benefit, as well as being aware of how and to whom to refer. Referral from a medical practitioner to a complementary practitioner has inherent difficulties in that, as certain therapies cannot always offer specific and predictable results, there is no specific therapy that is most effective for a specific disease or condition.

Although the medical profession has accepted the development of complementary therapies and seeks accommodation with it, complementary practitioners are still striving for state registration and national standards in order that complementary medicine may be integrated into the National Health Service and become more freely available.

Our health service may never be the same again as the link between traditional and complementary medicine forges these branches closer together. Already many hospitals, clinics and GP surgeries are incorporating the two systems together, in the interests of their patients.

For the complete accommodation of both concepts each professional, whether approaching the patient's health from a conventional or holistic point of view, must grow to appreciate the limitations of their own system in order to create a truly holistic health care system.

CHAPTER 2

Client management – the holistic approach

INTRODUCTION

Professional communication is a vital skill that helps to create a positive, trusting and co-operative therapeutic relationship between a therapist and a client. Holistic therapists need to have good communication skills in order to be able to identify client needs, desires and expectations of their chosen therapy treatment. Good communication allows a therapist to inform a client of the benefits of a chosen therapy, its limitations and the procedure involved in the delivery of the treatment service.

Professional communication involves the collection, recording and transmission of information for therapeutic benefit and will include assessing the client's health, their needs, treatment objectives and anticipated response. This chapter examines the importance of good client communication skills in order to establish a positive professional relationship with clients and to establish professional standards for the holistic therapy profession.

CLIENT COMMUNICATION SKILLS

When exchanging information during a consultation, therapists use four types of communication skills:

- speaking
- listening
- assessing non-verbal messages
- writing

Verbal Communication

Holistic therapy treatments involve one-to-one communication. The art of successful communication lies in **listening** to what the client is saying, **interpreting** the information being conveyed and giving **feedback** to verify the message has been received correctly.

Clients like to feel that their therapist is able to identify with their needs and that they have been listened to. When speaking to a client, it is important to choose words which convey intent clearly, concisely and tactfully and to avoid using language that the client may not understand, such as medical terminology.

Verbal communication involves co-operation from both the client and the therapist. When exchanging information, there should be periodic reflective pauses in the conversation. This provides opportunities to verify the message intended, and enables any corrections or alterations to be made.

Listening Skills

One of the most important skills in verbal communication is in the art of listening. Through effective listening a therapist can identify with client needs and customise a treatment plan.

> **KEY NOTE** Therapists should be aware that clients may not find it easy to make themselves understood. Depending on their condition, they may be speaking through a screen of emotionally-charged feelings. Effective listening will, therefore, involve understanding not only what the client is trying to say, but the tone and the emotion with which the information is imparted.

One of the main responsibilities of a therapist during a client consultation, is to help facilitate the client's communication and to concentrate on the focus of their message. **Active listening** should always be undertaken in a non-judgmental way. This will help the client feel safe to disclose sensitive and personal information in an honest and open way. To be non-judgmental, a therapist must withhold their own personal evaluation on the client's situation and respect the client's right to reveal their feelings in a supported environment.

It is important for therapists to realise that clients may be guarded about disclosing personal feelings until there is an established measure of trust. Therapists need to take care to consider their attitude and body language when carrying out a consultation, and should be aware of the importance of maintaining eye contact. Good listening skills require empathy and reflection. In other words, consider the client's feelings but also take time to reflect in order to avoid making incorrect assumptions, which would lead to inappropriate treatment planning and, ultimately, client dissatisfaction.

Barriers to Effective Communication

During a client consultation, it is useful to use a combination of **open-ended** and **closed questions**. Open-ended questions allow a client to reflect on their own feelings (e.g. 'What seems to be the trigger for your migraine attacks?' 'How do they make you feel?'), whilst closed questions are more focused on the specific client details (e.g. 'Are you taking any medication at the moment?'). Open-ended questions allow the client to give an answer in their own words; closed questions simply demand a yes or no response.

Therapists must take care not to suggest a client's response to a question or to finish sentences, both of which may block effective communication. In addition, it is important to keep the focus of the questions limited to the benefit of the treatment therapy session. Communication can be non-productive if the therapist is unable to set their own personal issues aside or if they make biased generalisations about their client's condition, assuming that they understand the problem.

If the therapist is obsessed with their own problems and they bring this into the therapy session, they will be unable to facilitate positive communication to the benefit of the client.

Non-verbal Communication

In order to enhance communication with clients, therapists need to consider the implications of non-verbal communication: messages that are projected by the body without the speaker's awareness. Non-verbal messages are an important part of communication as they often convey information about the emotional state of the client.

Non-verbal signs may include:
- **facial expressions** – lack of eye contact, frowning, grimacing
- **gestures** – gripping the sides of the chair or couch, fidgeting, nodding, making fists
- **sounds** – signs, grunts and groans, changes in breath, yawning
- **posture** – hunched shoulders
- **sudden movements** – looking down, tightening buttocks, toes lifting off the couch, lifting the head.

Therapists need to be aware of body language as a form of inner communication, and all non-verbal signs exhibited by a client should be observed throughout a consultation and treatment, and responded to in a positive way.

Therapists should also realise that, consciously or unconsciously, clients will be reading their body language. If the therapist behaves in an open and caring way, this will give the client a sense of security and shows that the therapist has sincerity in the professional relationship.

Written Communication

Written documentation is an important part of what establishes a holistic therapist as a professional practitioner. It confirms their educated assessment, choice of treatment and ongoing evaluation of the client's progress towards health and well-being.

Through written records, therapists can gain respect from others for their professional findings within the scope of their therapy. This can serve to increase the status and professionalism of the holistic therapy profession as a whole. Written records include the client consultation form, treatment plans, along with any referral data and correspondence from health care practitioners. Accurate records are important to help a therapist to recall specific details from previous treatments and to facilitate accurate, ongoing assessment and treatment planning. The systematic recording of specific information ensures the highest quality of therapeutic continuity and can protect a therapist from malpractice claims.

CLIENT CONSULTATION

Establishing trust during an initial consultation often results in client satisfaction and a continued therapeutic relationship, so it is important that sufficient time is allowed and the consultation is not rushed. It is important to ensure that the environment in which the consultation is to take place is as comfortable, private and warm as possible. If clients feel relaxed they are more likely to communicate openly, making it easier for the therapist to establish a rapport and identify their needs. It is also important to consider seating; sitting side by side may be less threatening and intimidating than sitting opposite.

A client consultation provides the foundation from which a suitable treatment plan may be formulated.

Consultations are necessary to:
- establish the parameters of a therapeutic and professional relationship
- gain the client's trust, respect and co-operation
- help put the client at ease, answer any queries and allay their fears about treatment
- help establish a client's medical history and to discuss their current state of health
- determine whether the client is suitable for treatment and whether they need to be referred to their GP or to other health care professionals
- determine the need for special care or adaptation of treatment, such as in the case of a pregnant client
- identify a client's needs, desires and expectations
- provide an opportunity for an explanation of the benefits, costs and limitations of the proposed treatment.

It is important when carrying out a consultation, that a client is assessed from a holistic point of view. Medical information is necessary for safety reasons, but it is equally important for the client's lifestyle, exercise, diet, occupation, stress levels and sleep patterns to be taken into consideration. This information will give a holistic view of a client's situation and may help to identify other factors which are relevant to the treatment plan and therapy proposed.

When asking personal questions, it is important for the therapist to maintain a polite and sensitive, but professional, manner. It should be stressed to clients that personal and medical questions are necessary in order for the therapist to establish how they can help.

If the consultation is carried out in a relaxed, rather than a formal, manner clients will be generally more co-operative with their answers. Forms are necessary as they form a structure for the consultation and may be used as a guide to ensure nothing is overlooked.

> **KEY NOTE** As there is no one form that meets the needs of all holistic therapies, a Consultation and Treatment Record form is provided within each therapy chapter of this book.

Visual Assessment

This aspect of the consultation begins when the therapist greets the client, observations may be made of the client's mood, their gait, posture and breathing pattern. Visual assessment may direct the therapist to any problems or any lifestyle enhancements which may benefit the client. It is important when making a visual assessment that therapists avoid diagnosing a condition – although they may recognise the signs and symptoms, only a medical practitioner may make a diagnosis. Within the limitations of their chosen therapy, therapists may observe and note specific signs, but should avoid labelling the condition.

If, upon assessing a client for treatment, a therapist suspects that the client may have a serious health problem, they should seek further clarification from the client's doctor before proceeding with the treatment.

Manual or Palpatory Assessment

This assessment is carried out through touch and is used to determine the condition of the soft tissues (skin, muscles, tendons, ligaments). Whatever modality of holistic therapy is being practised, therapists must be proficient in palpatory skills. By massaging, a therapist may be able to feel abnormalities in the tissues such as constrictions and adhesions, temperature changes and areas of excess fluid. Each holistic therapy requires a slightly different approach to palpation and abnormalities in the tissues or imbalances in energy flow may be determined by their characteristic feel within that discipline.

CONFIDENTIALITY

Confidentiality is an important part of the therapeutic relationship between a client and a therapist. Whilst carrying out a consultation it is important for a therapist to stress that all personal information relating to the client will remain completely confidential, and that information will not be disclosed to a third party without the client's written consent. Maintaining confidentiality projects a high degree of professionalism and prevents embarrassment and loss of client loyalty. It will also help to establish a good rapport with the client and encourages their confidence.

Therapists can maintain client confidentiality by:

- carrying out the consultation in private, or as privately as possible
- ensuring that all consultation and treatment records are stored in a secure place
- ensuring that client records and personal details are never left lying around
- never discussing a client's personal details or their treatment with another person, unless it is to liaise with another professional concerned with the client's progress, and the client's permission has been granted
- checking whether, if the client has to be contacted by phone, it is convenient to ring home or work, and when speaking to other parties that all details of their treatment remain private.

LIAISING WITH OTHER HEALTH CARE PROFESSIONALS

As the effectiveness of holistic therapies is increasingly proven, there are more and more opportunities for holistic therapists to work alongside health care professionals. Therapists must apply professional etiquette when liaising with other health care professionals and, if a client has been referred to them by another health care professional, they need to be able to write a status report on the client's progress.

Status Reports

Writing reports is an essential part of networking with other health care professionals. Status reports do not just report on an individual's progress they also raise awareness of the benefits of holistic therapies and demonstrate their value in health care generally.

A status report should include the following information:

- a general introduction explaining how the client was referred
- a summary of the client's main presenting problem or problems
- the therapist's findings
- the therapeutic modalities used and their results
- the therapist's evaluation of client progress
- recommendations as to which therapy, or combination of therapy treatments, would be required to maintain progress.

Referral

It is also necessary for therapists to be able to refer a client to a medical or other health care professional if they present with a contra-indication or medical condition requiring medical care. It is best for the therapist to have a pre-prepared form for this purpose. Use headed note paper, and a form layout which states clearly and concisely what information is required (see page 10). This may either be taken by the client to their doctor or may be posted with a stamped addressed envelope. It is advisable to include with the referral form, literature on the therapy proposed, in order to raise the doctor's awareness of its methodology and potential benefits.

It is important that therapists make it clear that, when referring a client to their doctor, they are not asking the doctor to take responsibility for the therapeutic treatment. They are seeking more information or advice regarding the client's medical state in order to decide the client's suitability for treatment.

Example of Referral Form

Therapist's Name
Clinic Address
Date

Doctor's Name _____

Surgery Address _____

Holistic therapy treatment for which medical referral is required

_____

Dear Doctor _____ ,

I am writing with regard to one of your patients   (*Patient's name*)   of

(*Patient's address*) _____

who has requested (*Type of treatment*) treatment. _____

(*Enter explanation of treatment and its benefits*)_____

_____

_____

I have carried out a detailed consultation with this patient and would be grateful if you could outline any recommendations or restrictions that you would advise regarding their medical suitability to the proposed treatment by completing the consent form below.
Should you require any further information regarding the proposed treatment, please do not hesitate to contact me.
Thank you for your assistance in this matter

(*Therapist's name and signature*)   _____

Doctor's consent
I agree/disagree that the proposed treatment of   _____
would be suitable/unsuitable for this patient.
I recommend the following restrictions.

_____

_____

_____

Signed:_____   Name: _____

PROFESSIONALISM

Professional standards are the guidelines set in order to promote the integrity, scope of practice and professionalism of holistic therapies. They reflect current educational standards and are determined by professional associations. As the holistic therapy profession experiences growing demand, there is a greater need for distinct borders and standards to be defined as these will help to distinguish it from other health care professions and to establish it as a profession in its own right.

Professional Ethics

Professional ethics reflect the professional standards and moral principles that govern an individual or group's course of action and behaviour. All professional associations in this field publish their own code of ethics that their members are required to follow.

Typical ethics guidelines for holistic therapists are as follows:
- Acknowledge contra-indications for holistic therapies, and refer to the appropriate health professional before any treatment is given.
- Accurately inform clients, members of the public and other health care professionals of the scope and limitations of the therapy or therapies practised.
- Have commitment to the industry by providing the highest quality of service to clients at all times.
- Represent the industry honestly by only providing services in which you are qualified to practice.
- Have respect for the religious, spiritual, social or political views of the client, irrespective of creed, race, colour or sex.
- Never discriminate against other clients, therapists or other health care professionals.
- Act in a co-operative manner with other health care professionals and refer cases which are out of the sphere of the therapy field in which you practice.
- Always present a professional image by practising the highest standards of personal and salon or clinic hygiene.
- Conduct yourself in a professional manner at all times, with honesty and integrity.
- Be courteous to clients and treat them with dignity and respect.
- Keep accurate, up to date records of client treatment, including advice given and the outcome or outcomes.
- Safeguard the confidentiality of all client information, unless disclosure is required by law. If liaison is required with a health care professional, the client's written permission must be sought.
- Only provide treatment when there is reasonable expectations that it will be advantageous to the client.
- Ensure that working premises comply with all current health, safety and hygiene legislation.
- Never give unqualified advice.
- Never diagnose a medical condition or injury.

- Never prescribe or advise on the use of medication.
- Maintain and improve professional development through continuing education and personal development.
- Never abuse the client–therapist relationship.
- Explain the treatment accurately to the client and discuss the fees involved before any treatment commences.
- Ensure that any advertising is accurate, reflects the professionalism of the industry and that it does not contravene any consumer legislation.
- Be adequately insured to practice the therapy or therapies in which you are qualified.

SETTING PROFESSIONAL BOUNDARIES

In order to have a healthy and professional relationship with clients there should be a balance between care and compassion for each client, and maintaining a distance. The setting of boundaries provides an important foundation upon which to build a professional relationship with the client. Clients need to be given space to facilitate healing in a therapeutic relationship, and it is, therefore, important that a therapist avoids bringing items on their own agenda into the treatment room.

Transference and Counter-transference

There is always a risk of **transference** in a client–therapist relationship. This means that the client begins to personalise the professional relationship and, thus, steps over the professional boundary. There is also a risk of **counter-transference** when a therapist has difficulty in maintaining a professional distance from the client's problems and begins to assume a friend or counsellor role.

If either of these situations occur, it is important for the therapist to realise how potentially damaging this can be for the client and how it detracts from their healing process. If therapists are unable to keep a healthy distance from a client and their problems, they need to consider whether the drive to help the client beyond their professional boundary may be fulfilling a need in them that is not being met elsewhere. If this need is not met and the problem continues to go unaddressed, it may also affect future therapeutic relationships.

CHAPTER 3

Pathological conditions – a guide for the holistic therapist

INTRODUCTION

As growth and interest in holistic therapies continues to increase, there are more and more people seeking help from a holistic therapist for their emotional and physical well-being.

Holistic therapists, therefore, need to be knowledgeable within the sphere of their chosen therapy and must be able to communicate effectively with other health care professionals. These skills help the therapist to assess the health and condition of their client before treatment is commenced.

In order to become an accepted and respected member of holistic health care teams, it is vital that therapists equip themselves with a sound underpinning knowledge of clinical conditions in order to be able to assess:
- whether the client needs to be referred to their GP
- whether the client may be contra-indicated for treatment
- how a client's condition may affect or restrict their proposed treatment.

The therapist must be able to make an informed decision as to a suitable treatment plan that is within safe and ethical medical guidelines.

It is very important that a therapist never diagnoses a client's medical condition and always refers the client to their GP for clarification of their medical condition before any form of treatment is commenced.

This chapter is designed as a quick reference guide to some of the common pathological conditions which a therapist may encounter in their daily work, and the precautions and restrictions they may present on treatments proposed.

> **KEY NOTE** Whilst the information given in the following section is an accurate representation of each condition in generic terms, all clients will vary in the severity of their condition. Each client should be assessed individually at the time of the proposed treatment and re-assessed on subsequent treatments. Since this is a general guide, therapists are encouraged to seek further clarification of a client's medical condition from the GP and from the client themselves.

ALPHABETICAL LIST OF COMMON CONDITIONS

Acne Vulgaris

A common inflammatory disorder of the sebaceous glands which leads to the overproduction of sebum. It involves the face, back and chest and is characterised by the presence of comedones, papules, and in more severe cases cysts and scars. Acne Vulgaris is primarily androgen induced, appearing most frequently at puberty and usually persisting for a considerable period of time.

Cautions, Restrictions and Recommendations

- Acne is not contagious and can not be spread from one area of the body to another. However, if there is extensive inflammation avoid treatment in the affected area.
- Clients suffering with acne may have a low self-esteem due to its appearance and may benefit psychologically from holistic therapies.

AIDS

A viral infection that progressively destroys the immunity of the individual. It is caused by the **Human Immunodeficiency Virus** (HIV) which primarily affects the T-lymphocytes, resulting in the suppression of the body's immune response. AIDS patients become vulnerable to infections that only produce mild symptoms in other people. They may also be prone to cancers.

HIV infection is caused by contact with infected blood or body fluids. It is common in drug addicts who may be using infected injection needles and syringes and can be contracted through having unprotected sexual intercourse. It is more prevalent in homosexuals. Remember Haemophiliacs are prone to have AIDS due to infected blood from transfusions.

Cautions, Restrictions and Recommendations

- It is a matter of personal choice for a therapist in deciding whether to treat a client with AIDS. Although it is recommended that protective gloves are worn, some therapists may feel that this is inappropriate since it is the power of human touch that underpins holistic therapies.

- Refrain from treating a client with AIDS if you or they have an open wound.
- Relaxation therapies of short duration may be of benefit.
- Ensure that the client is not exposed to any form of infection.
- Special precautions have to be taken if the client has other associated diseases, such as tuberculosis, herpes or hepatitis B.

Angina

Angina is pain in the left side of the chest which usually radiates to the left arm. It is caused by an insufficient blood supply to the heart muscle; attacks usually occur on exertion or excitement. The pain is often described as constricting or suffocating, and can last for a few seconds or longer. Patient may become pale and sweaty. This condition indicates ischaemic heart disease.

Cautions, Restrictions and Recommendations

- As stress predisposes an angina attack, massage and other relaxation therapies can help by reducing stress levels. These techniques reduce the activity of the sympathetic nervous system which is partly responsible for coronary vasoconstriction.
- As sudden exposure to extreme heat or cold can bring on an attack, keep the client warm and avoid extreme fluctuations in temperature.
- It is important that clients have their necessary medications with them when they attend for treatment, as they may need it in the event of an emergency.

Ankylosing Spondylitis

This is a systemic joint disease characterised by inflammation of the intervertebral disc spaces, costo-vertebral and sacroiliac joints. Fibrosis, calcification, ossification and stiffening of joints are common and the spine becomes rigid. Typically, clients complain of persistent or intermittent lower back pain. Kyphosis is present when the thoracic or cervical regions of the spine are affected and the weight of the head compresses the vertebrae and bends the spine forward. This condition can cause muscular atrophy, loss of balance and falls. Typically, Ankylosing spondylitis affects young, male adults.

Cautions, Restrictions and Recommendations

- Position the client so that they feel most comfortable – extra cushioning and support may be required.
- Avoid forcibly mobilising ankylosed joints and, in the case of cervical spondylitis, avoid hyperextending the neck.
- Gentle massage to the back and limbs may be very beneficial as the heat generated may help to ease the pain.
- Advise the client to do breathing exercises regularly in order to help mobilise the thorax.

Anxiety

This can be defined as a fear of the unknown. As an illness, it can vary from a mild form to panic attacks and severe phobias that can be disabling socially, psychologically and, at times, physically. It presents with feelings of dread that something serious is likely to happen, is associated with palpitations, rapid breathing, sweaty hands, tremor (shakiness), dry mouth, general indigestion, a feeling of butterflies in the stomach, occasional diarrhoea and generalised aches and pains in the muscles. It can present with similar features to mild or moderate depression of the agitated type. Anxiety is associated with genetic and behavioural predisposition, and can be caused by a traumatic experience or physical illness, i.e. hyperthyroidism.

Cautions, Restrictions and Recommendations

- Clients are likely to present with variable symptoms and, therefore, a thorough assessment is required.
- Relaxation exercises and holistic therapies are likely to be a valuable source of help.
- Clients with anxiety are more likely to become emotionally dependent on their therapist; therapists need to be aware of this possibility and may need to refer the client to another practitioner.

Arthritis – Gout

This is a joint disorder due to uric acid crystals accumulating in the joint cavity. It commonly affects the peripheral joints, commonly the metatarsophalangeal joint of the big toe. Kidneys can also be affected and other cartilage may be involved, including the ear pinna.

Cautions, Restrictions and Recommendations

- Avoid massaging during the acute stages – the affected joint should be rested due to inflammation.
- In the sub-acute phase light massage may be carried out in the surrounding areas.
- In the chronic stages light to medium massage may be carried out in order to help increase the circulation and the elimination of uric acid crystals.

Arthritis – Osteoarthritis

This is a joint disease characterised by the breakdown of articular cartilage, the growth of bony spikes and the swelling of the surrounding synovial membrane, leading to stiffness and tenderness of the joint. Is also known as degenerative arthritis. It is common in the elderly and takes a progressive course.

This condition involves varying degrees of joint pain, stiffness, limitation of movement, joint instability and deformity. It commonly affects the weight bearing joints – the hips, knees, the lumbar and cervical vertebrae.

Cautions, Restrictions and Recommendations

- Passive and gentle friction movements around the joint may be beneficial where there is minimal pain, but excessive movement may cause joint pain and damage.

- Gentle massage may help with muscle spasms, joint stiffness and muscle atrophy.
- Always ask the client to demonstrate the range of possible movement at each joint as this will show you where the limitations of treatment are.

Arthritis – Rheumatoid

Rheumatoid arthritis causes chronic inflammation of peripheral joints, resulting in pain, stiffness and potential damage to joints. It can cause severe disability. Joint swellings and rheumatoid nodules are tender.

Cautions, Restrictions and Recommendations

- Although holistic therapies cannot cure arthritis, they can help to prevent its progress by promoting relaxation and reducing discomfort.
- In the early stages of diagnosis, clients should be encouraged to have treatment in order to maintain the range of joint movements and to help prevent contractures.
- In the acute stage, avoid massaging but encourage passive movement of the affected joints.
- In the chronic stage gentle effleurage, petrissage and friction movements can help to reduce the thickening that occurs in and around the articular cartilage.
- Always ensure there is no pain and that care is taken when gently mobilising a joint.
- Treatment is generally of shorter duration as clients may be taking pain killers and may be unable to give adequate feedback.

Asthma

Asthma attacks range from shortness of breath to great difficulty in breathing. It is due to spasm or swelling of the bronchial tubes, caused by hypersensitivity to allergens such as pollen, pet hair, dust mites, and various proteins in foodstuffs such as shellfish, eggs and milk. Asthma may be exacerbated by exercise, anxiety, stress or smoking. It runs in families and can be associated with hayfever and eczema.

Cautions, Restrictions and Recommendations

- Always obtain a detailed history during the consultation stage, specifically the triggers that bring on an attack. If the client has a history of allergies, ensure they are not allergic to any preparations or substances you are proposing to use.
- Relaxation treatments and deep breathing exercises can help to reduce bronchiospasm and should be encouraged.
- Position the clients according to their individual comfort, usually in a semi-reclined position.
- It is advisable for the client to have their medication to hand, in the event of an attack.

ATHEROSCLEROSIS

This is a circulatory system condition characterised by a thickening, narrowing, hardening and loss of elasticity of the walls of the arteries.

Cautions, Restrictions and Recommendations

■ Clients with atherosclerosis are prone to thrombus formation. Using deeper manipulation could encourage any thrombus to dislodge and travel to the lungs, heart or the brain. This could cause serious problems such as a heart attack or stroke.

■ See **Thrombosis**.

■ Refer the client to their GP if they have a history of previous strokes, heart attack, angina or thrombosis and, if treatment is encouraged, use gentle techniques and avoid over stimulation.

Bronchitis

Bronchitis is a chronic or acute inflammation of the bronchial tubes. Chronic bronchitis is common in smokers and may lead to emphysema, which is caused by damage to the lung structure. Acute bronchitis can result from a recent cold or flu.

Cautions, Restrictions and Recommendations

■ Take care when positioning clients with bronchitis; if it is possible for the treatment, it is advisable to position the client with their head elevated higher than their feet with the use of props and pillows.

■ Encourage the client to breathe slowly and deeply throughout the treatment.

■ Sufferers of chronic bronchitis are prone to respiratory infection. Such clients should not receive treatment from therapists who have even the mildest form of acute chest infection which they could pass on.

Cancer of the Bladder

This cancer usually presents with blood in the urine and with urgency and pain on passing urine. Secondary symptoms may arise if it has spread to the lungs, liver, lymph nodes and neighbouring tissues.

Cautions, Restrictions and Recommendations

■ Consult the client's GP or consultant regarding the extent of the disease.

■ If indicated, a light massage of short duration, avoiding the abdomen, may be beneficial.

Cancer of the Breast

Most breast cancers are detected when the client notices a breast or axillary lump; mammography screening can confirm a diagnosis. Breast cancer can present as redness and pain, discharge from or retraction of the nipple. Cancer can spread locally to the axilla and neck lymph nodes, causing oedema of the arm, or by blood to the lungs, bone and liver. The type of breast cancer can determine whether the spread is rapid or very slow.

Cautions, Restrictions and Recommendations

■ Consult the client's GP or consultant regarding the extent of the disease, especially if a hard mass is felt under the axilla or in the chest wall.

■ It is a controversial issue as to whether massage can contribute to the spread of cancer. The spread of cancer is also determined by the type (some spread rapidly while others are slow growing).

■ Avoid areas of exposure to radiation if the client is having radiotherapy treatment.

■ Radio and chemotherapy can reduce the client's immunity and, therefore, you should avoid massaging if you have an infection.

■ Clients who have had surgery that involved removal of the axillary nodes are likely to have oedema of the arm. Provided permission has been granted by the client's GP or consultant, elevate the oedematous arm above heart level throughout the massage. Gently massage the arm with strokes directed towards the axilla. Advise the client to open and close the hand tightly six to eight times every few hours (the contraction of the muscles will help venous and lymphatic flow).

Cancer of the Cervix

Cervical cancer is asymptomatic in the early stages. Later there may be foul-smelling, blood-stained discharge through the vagina. Lower back pain, loss of weight, unexplained anaemia and pain during intercourse are other symptoms.

Cautions, Restrictions and Recommendations

■ Consult the client's GP or consultant to find out about the extent of the disease and the form of treatment the client is undergoing.

■ If the client is receiving radiation treatment, remember that their general immunity may be depressed and exposure to any type of infection should be avoided.

■ Advise all clients to have regular smear tests as recommended by their GP or specialist.

Cancer of the Colon

In the early stages, the signs and symptoms are vague and are related to the location of the cancer. A dull abdominal pain may or may not be present. General symptoms include loss of weight, fatigue, anaemia and weakness.

If the tumour is on the right side of the abdomen (caecum or ascending colon), symptoms of obstruction appear slowly. Tumours in this region tend to spread along the walls of the gut, without narrowing the lumen. If the tumour is on the left side (descending colon, sigmoid colon or rectum), the signs of obstruction appear early in the disease. There may be constipation or diarrhoea with passage of pencil-shaped or ribbon-like stools. The blood in the stools may be red or dark in colour.

Cautions, Restrictions and Recommendations

■ Consult the client's GP or consultant regarding the spread of the disease and the type of treatment.

■ If massage is indicated, a light massage of short duration is recommended, avoiding the abdominal area.

Cancer of the Gall Bladder

Indigestion and colicky pain may be present, especially after a fatty meal. The pain is located in the upper right quadrant of the abdomen and may be referred to the back, the right shoulder, right scapula or between the scapula.

Cautions, Restrictions and Recommendations

- Consult the client's GP or consultant regarding the spread of the disease and the type of treatment.
- If massage is indicated, a light massage of short duration is recommended, avoiding the upper right quadrant of the abdominal cavity.

Cancer of the Kidney

There are no symptoms initially. Subsequently, symptoms include a swelling in the abdomen; blood in the urine denotes advanced disease. Encourage a client to consult their GP if they complain of blood in their urine.

Cautions, Restrictions and Recommendations

- Consult the client's GP or consultant regarding the extent of the disease and the type of treatment.
- If the client is undergoing chemotherapy, remember that their immunity will be reduced – do not offer treatment if you are suffering from any infection.
- If indicated, massage may be beneficial in reducing the leg cramps that can be a common symptom of this condition – a light soothing massage is recommended.

Cancer of the Liver

The more common type of liver cancer is one which has spread from other areas of the body – metastatic carcinoma. Spread commonly occurs from those parts of the body which supply blood to the liver (the stomach, intestine and pancreas for example). Cancer can also arise in the liver tissue itself – primary cancer.

Liver cancer may be present as a swelling in the upper right quadrant of the abdomen and is associated with jaundice or fluid in the abdomen. Other general symptoms may include weight loss, weakness, loss of appetite.

This type of cancer is usually well advanced when diagnosed, whether arising from the liver or secondary to cancer elsewhere in the body.

Cautions, Restrictions and Recommendations

- Consult the client's GP or consultant as to the extent of disease and the type of treatment.
- If massage is indicated, a light massage of short duration and avoiding the abdominal area may be beneficial.

- If the client is having chemotherapy or radiation treatment, remember that their immunity will be lowered and avoid massaging if you are harbouring any type of infection.

Cancer of the Lung

Lung cancer may be caused by chronic inhalation of cancer-producing air and industrial pollutants, such as cigarette smoke, asbestos fibres etc. There are no initial symptoms and usually it is detected only in the advanced stages. Late symptoms include chronic cough, hoarseness, difficulty in breathing, chest pain, blood in the sputum, weight loss and weakness.

Cautions, Restrictions and Recommendations

- The benefits of massage in reducing stress levels in these individuals is undisputed. However, massage may help to spread the cancer to other regions, especially if it has already spread to lymph nodes or other neighbouring structures.
- Consult the client's GP or consultant as to the extent of the disease and the type of treatment.
- If the client is receiving radiation or chemotherapy treatment avoid massaging over radiation sites and remember their immunity is reduced.

Cancer – Oral

This may be caused by chronic irritation of the mucosa of the oral cavity, as in tobacco chewing. Recurrence of chronic ulcers in the mouth can also lead to this type of cancer. Oral cancer may appear as a non-healing, slow-growing, red ulcer or as a growth. Usually it is painful and firm to touch.

Cautions, Restrictions and Recommendations

- Consult the client's GP or consultant as to the extent of the disease and the type of treatment.
- This type of cancer can spread to the lymph nodes of the neck. The nodes are felt as hard, rounded or irregular swellings. Treatment is with radiation or surgery.
- Radiation treatment lowers the immunity in the local area and these individuals are prone to thrush and dental caries.
- Avoid massage to the face and neck.
- Encourage the client to stop smoking and drinking.

Cancer of the Ovaries

This cancer is asymptomatic until the late stages. Diagnosis is usually made after the cancer has spread extensively. The symptoms are vague and are usually associated with gastrointestinal problems such as bloating of the abdomen, mild abdominal pain and excessive passage of gas. There may be fluid in the peritoneal cavity in late stages. Hormone changes may result in abnormal vaginal bleeding.

Cautions, Restrictions and Recommendations

■ Consult the client's GP or consultant as to the extent of the disease and the type of treatment.

■ If massage is indicated, a light massage of short duration, avoiding the abdomen is recommended.

■ Remember that immunity is suppressed in a client who is receiving radiation or chemotherapy – avoid massage if you are harbouring any type of infection.

Cancer of the Pancreas

The patient presents with severe weight loss and pain in the lower back. The pain increases a few hours after taking food and becomes worse on lying down. If the tumour is growing around the bile duct, obstruction may result in jaundice and diarrhoea. The accumulation of bilirubin under the skin causes severe itching. The jaundice may be so severe that the skin may turn green or black as the bilirubin changes in structure.

The associated reduction in bile slows down the absorption and digestion of fat, causing clay-coloured, foul-smelling stools and diarrhoea.

The cancer spreads directly and rapidly to the surrounding tissues including the lymph nodes and liver. Kidneys, spleen and blood vessels may also be involved. The symptoms may vary according to the tissues affected.

Cautions, Restrictions and Recommendations

■ This type of cancer spreads rapidly and massage could spread the cancer further. However, often this cancer is diagnosed at an advanced stage when the condition cannot be worsened.

■ Consult the client's GP or consultant as to the extent of the disease and the type of treatment.

■ If massage is indicated, a light massage of short duration may be suitable. Avoid the abdominal area if the disease is in an advanced stage.

Cancer of the Prostate

Usually no symptoms are seen. If the cancer is located close to the urethra, there may be a frequency of micturition, urgency, difficulty in voiding, blood in urine or blood in the ejaculate. Cancer of the prostate is often diagnosed by rectal examination, where it feels nodular and hard. Prostate cancer usually spreads to the bones and produces bony pain. Weakness of the bone may lead to fractures after trivial injury. In the advanced stage, as in all cancers, the person loses weight and is anaemic.

Cautions, Restrictions and Recommendations

■ Consult the client's GP or consultant to determine the stage of the disease.

■ If massage is indicated, a light massage of short duration may be beneficial.

Cancer of the Skin

Basal cell carcinomas are of different types and can occur as pinkish, smooth swellings with blood vessels over the lesion. They can also ulcerate. Common sites of basal cell carcinoma are: the side of the nose, naso-labial area, around the eyes, temple and front of the ear. Sometimes these cancers appear as thickened areas of skin on the chest and back that are lightly pigmented. Squamous cell carcinoma appears as a palpable swelling that grows slowly.

Melanomas are common on the head, neck and leg areas and usually arise from pre-existing, pigmented areas, such as a darkish mole. These appear as irregular growths that may be blue, red, white or pigmented. Melanomas are usually associated with itching, can ulcerate or bleed and have a tender base.

Cautions, Restrictions and Recommendations

- Consult the GP or consultant regarding massage of individuals who have been diagnosed with skin cancer. You need to know about the mode and spread of the disease.
- Treatment varies according to the type and stage of cancer.

Cancer of the Stomach

In the early stages, the person has chronic pain or discomfort in the upper part of the abdomen. Since the symptoms are vague, this cancer is often not diagnosed until it has spread considerably. There is weight loss, anaemia, loss of appetite and the person will feel easily fatigued. Vomiting is common and often the contents contain blood. A mass may be felt in the upper abdomen. Indigestion and acidity is not relieved by medication.

Cautions, Restrictions and Recommendations

- Consult the client's GP or consultant as to the extent of the disease and the type of treatment.
- This type of cancer spreads rapidly through the bloodstream and lymphatic system. Therefore, there may be a risk that massage could perpetuate the spread of the disease.
- If the client has had radiation treatment or surgery, avoid the affected site.
- Remember that radiation reduces immunity.
- Do not massage if you have even a mild infection.

Cancer – Testis

A slight enlargement of the testis is the first symptom. It may be accompanied by pain, discomfort and heaviness of the scrotum. Soon there is a rapid enlargement of the testis which can become hot and red.

Cautions, Restrictions and Recommendations

- Consult the client's GP or consultant as to the extent of the disease. If confined only to the testis, a light, soothing, whole body massage may be beneficial.

Carpal Tunnel Syndrome

Characterised by pain and numbness in the thumb or hand, this condition results from pressure on the median nerve of the wrist. Pain and a pins-and-needles sensation may radiate to the elbow. It is known to cause severe pain at night and can cause muscle wasting of the hand. There is a higher risk of this condition in occupations requiring repetitive strains of the wrist, such as massage therapists and secretaries.

Cautions, Restrictions and Recommendations

■ Avoid localised massage to the wrist if there is acute inflammation present in the area.
■ In a chronic condition, this condition can be helped by elevating the limb to encourage lymph drainage, localised massage to loosen scar tissue and passively moving the elbow, wrist and fingers in order to maintain the range of movement. It is also important to massage the neck, shoulders and arms in order to help to relieve discomfort.
■ It is important to help the client to identify the risk factors associated with this condition and to explore ways in which they can be avoided.
■ Clients may need to discuss their situation with an occupational health advisor in their place of work, if one is available.
■ Remedial exercises, such as passive stretching of the flexors and extensors of the wrist, can be helpful in aiding this condition.

Congenital Heart Disease

This is a defect in the formation of the heart which usually decreases its efficiency. Defects may result in non-closure of the opening between the right and left ventricle (ventricular septal defects); non-closure of the opening between the right and left atrium (atrial septal defect); narrowing of the aorta (coaraction of the aorta); narrowing of the pulmonary artery (pulmonary stenosis); non-closure of the communication between the pulmonary artery and the aorta that exists in the foetus until delivery (patent ductus arteriosus); or a combination of defects. The symptoms may vary according to the severity of the defect.

Cautions, Restrictions and Recommendations

■ Always take a detailed history of the client's symptoms and medical or surgical treatment.
■ It is important to seek clearance from the client's GP before treating as they may advise on the nature and duration of the proposed treatment.
■ In general, massage and other associated therapies may be beneficial due to relaxation, although a treatment of short duration is often recommended.
■ Depending on the type of defect and surgery undertaken, it may be more appropriate and comfortable for the client to be treated in a seated position.

Contact Dermatitis

Dermatitis literally means inflammation of the skin. Contact dermatitis is the result of a primary irritant which causes the skin to become red, dry and inflamed. Substances which are likely to cause this reaction include acids, alkalis, solvent, perfumes, lanolin, detergent and nickels. There may be skin infection as well.

Cautions, Restrictions and Recommendations

- Always take a detailed history of this condition and ask about any chemicals the client is allergic to.
- With clients who have a history of allergies, always test a small area of skin with the proposed substances to be used in the treatment. Watch for itching, redness and swelling.
- If a reaction is positive, wash the area immediately. If the reaction is severe, refer the client to their GP.
- Avoid treating an area which is red, sore and inflamed. There is a risk of increasing the inflammation and introducing infection.

Cystitis

This is an inflammation of the urinary bladder, usually caused by infection of the bladder lining. Common symptoms are pain just above the pubic bone, lower back or inner thigh, blood in the urine, and frequent, urgent and painful urination.

Cautions, Restrictions and Recommendations

- It is important to encourage a client to increase their intake of fluids (water and cranberry juice). If symptoms persist, they may need GP advice and assessment.
- Massage over the lower abdomen is best avoided to reduce the chances of causing pain and spasm induction.

Depression

This combines symptoms of lowered mood, loss of appetite, poor sleep, lack of concentration and interest, lack of sense of enjoyment, occasional constipation and loss of libido. There may be occasions of suicidal thinking, death wish or active suicidal attempts. Depression can be the result of chemical imbalance, usually related to serotonin and noradrenalin. The cause of depression could be endogenous if there is no obvious reason for the condition. It is thought also to be linked to genetic predisposition, may be the result of a physical illness, of the actual loss of a close relative, object, limb or loss of a relationship.

A depressed person usually looks miserable, hunchbacked, downcast and may avoid eye contact. The severity of the condition can be variable, but if very severe, may become psychotic manifested by hallucinations, delusions, paranoia or thought disorders.

Cautions, Restrictions and Recommendations

- A depressed client can present with physical ailments including backache, gastro-intestinal symptoms (usually constipation) and headaches.
- Physical illness can present with depression. These might include long-term illness, terminal illness, Parkinson's disease and arthritis, for instance.

■ Therapists must try to ensure that clients do not become emotionally dependent. They may need to be referred to another practitioner.

■ At any time, if there is any inclination to suicidal thinking, the client should be referred to their GP.

■ Holistic therapies, in particular the effects of certain essential oils with aromatherapy massage, are well known to help clients cope with depression.

Diabetes Mellitus

This is a carbohydrate metabolism disorder that results from inadequate production or use of insulin by the pancreas.

There are two types of diabetes:

1. **Insulin Dependent**, **Type I** or **Juvenile-Onset Diabetes**. This is thought to be caused by genetic predisposition. People with Type I diabetes have little or no ability to produce the hormone insulin and are entirely dependent on insulin injections to sustain life.

2. **Non-Insulin Dependent**, **Type II** or **Maturity-Onset Diabetes**. This is more common in those who are overweight and usually occurs after the age of 40. In this type of diabetes the pancreas retains some ability to produce insulin but this is inadequate for the body's needs. Patients may require treatment with oral hypoglycaemic drugs. In both types of diabetes the diet should be carefully controlled, with adequate carbohydrates. An imbalance in the diet and in the amount of insulin leads to hypoglycaemia.

Remember that diabetes of any type can cause damage to the eye retina, kidneys, peripheral nerves and can be associated with ischaemic heart disease.

Cautions, Restrictions and Recommendations

■ Always take a detailed history and liaise with the client's GP to find out which type of diabetes the client is suffering from.

■ It has been indicated that holistic therapies may have an effect on daily insulin levels. Therefore, close monitoring should be undertaken.

■ It is important for the therapist to be aware that feedback may be inadequate in those with decreased sensation (resulting from nerve damage). Therefore, pressure used in treatments should be carefully monitored.

■ Caution should be exercised – diabetic clients may have acute complications such as hypoglycaemia resulting in dizziness, weakness, pallor, rapid heart beat and excessive sweating.

■ Always ensure that the client brings their glucose and other medication when coming for treatment.

Eczema

Eczema is a mild to chronic inflammatory skin condition characterised by itchiness, redness and the presence of small blisters that may be dry or weep if the surface is scratched. Eczema is noncontagious; one cause may be genetic, due to internal or external influences. It can cause scaly and thickened skin mainly at flexures, e.g. cubital area of the elbows and the back of the knees.

Cautions, Restrictions and Recommendations
- Try and identify the causes and factors which may increase irritation or inflammation.
- Avoid any topical application which may exacerbate the condition.
- If the condition is stress-induced, massage and associated therapies may help in stress reduction.
- Avoid contact with inflamed areas and treat as a localised contra-indication.

Epilepsy
This is a neurological disorder that makes the individual susceptible to recurrent and temporary seizures. Epilepsy is a complex condition and classification of types of epilepsy are not definitive. However, four basic types are recognised:

1. **Generalised** – this may take the form of major or tonic–clonic seizures (formerly known as *grand mal*) At the onset the patient falls to the ground unconscious with their muscles in a state of spasm (tonic phase). This is followed by convulsive movements (the clonic phase) when the tongue may be bitten and urinary incontinence may occur. Movements gradually cease and the patient may rouse in a state of confusion, complaining of a headache or may fall asleep.

2. **Partial** – this may be idiopathic or a symptom of structural damage to the brain. In one type of partial idiopathic epilepsy, often affecting children, seizures may take the form of absences (formerly known as *petit mal*), in which there are brief spells of unconsciousness lasting for a few seconds. The eyes stare blankly and there may be fluttering movements of the lids and momentary twitching of the fingers and mouth. This form of epilepsy seldom appears before the age of three or after adolescence. It often subsides spontaneously in adult life, but may be followed by the onset of generalised or partial epilepsy.

3. **Focal** – this is partial epilepsy due to brain damage (either local or due to a stroke). The nature of the seizure depends on the location of the damage in the brain. In a Jacksonian motor seizure, the convulsive movements may spread from the thumb to the hand, arm and face.

4. **Psychomotor** – this type of epilepsy is caused by a dysfunction in the cortex of the temporal lobe of the brain. Symptoms may include hallucinations of smell, taste, sight and hearing. Throughout the attack, the patient is in a state of clouded awareness and afterwards may have no recollection of the event.

Cautions, Restrictions and Recommendations
- Always refer to the client's GP regarding type and nature of epilepsy that the client suffers from.
- If on controlled medication, the chances of seizure are minimal. However, caution is advised due to the complexity of this condition.
- It has never been reported that holistic therapies have provoked the onset of epilepsy. However, there is a theoretical risk in that deep relaxation or over stimulation could provoke an attack (although this has never been proven in practice).

Fibromyalgia

This chronic condition produces musculo-skeletal pain. Predominant symptoms include widespread musculo-skeletal pain, lethargy and fatigue. Other characteristic features include a non-refreshing sleep pattern in which the patient feels exhausted and more tired when they wake than later in the day, and interrupted sleep. Other recognised symptoms include early morning stiffness, pins-and-needles sensation, unexplained headaches, poor concentration, memory loss, low mood, urinary frequency, abdominal pain, irritable bowel syndrome. Anxiety and depression are also common.

Cautions, Restrictions and Recommendations

- Avoid deep massage on localised tender areas.
- Caution is advised regarding stiffness.
- Relaxation is integral to reduce muscle spasm and reduce feelings of stress.

Gall Stones

A gall stone is a hard mass composed of bile pigments, cholesterol and calcium salts which forms in the gall bladder. Gall stones may exist for many years without causing symptoms. However, they may cause pain, or may pass into the common bile duct and cause an obstruction to the flow of bile into the duodenum. Symptoms range from recurring colicky pain the right upper abdomen to indigestion and signs of a tender liver area, with jaundice.

Cautions, Restrictions and Recommendations

- Avoid massage to the upper right quadrant of the abdomen.

Hay Fever

An allergic reaction involving the mucous passages of the upper respiratory tract and the conjunctiva of the eyes, caused by pollen or other allergens. Symptoms include nose blockages, sneezing and watery eyes.

Cautions, Restrictions and Recommendations

- Keep a detailed history of the allergy.
- Keep your treatment areas dust free, ensure proper ventilation and air conditioning.
- Avoid or minimise the presence of flowering plants.

Headache

This is general pain which affects the head, excluding facial pain. It can result from diseases affecting ear, nose and throat, e.g. sinusitis, as well as eye problems which can be corrected by glasses.

There are various types of headache:

1. **Simple headache** – this may occur at times of stress, during menstrual periods, the day after heavy alcohol consumption or as part of cold and flu symptoms. These are transient and normally settle spontaneously. At most they require simple analgesia.
2. **Chronic headache** – includes daily headache and tension headache. The pain can be severe and disabling. It may affect the whole head, behind the eyes or may be just a frontal headache. The client often describes the pain as 'like a band around the head'.

3. **Headache due to radiation from cervical spines (Cervicalgia)** – this is normally felt in the back and sides of the head and can present with neck pain.
4. **Migraine headache** – see Migraine.
5. **Headache due to intracranial (inside brain) disease** – this type of headache can present with nausea and vomiting and may cause other neurological signs and symptoms. It is symptomatic of a brain tumour for example.

Cautions, Restrictions and Recommendations
- Any type of therapy which can reduce stress will help to relieve headaches.
- Muscular relaxation is an important part of therapy.
- Remember that any long-lasting headache should be assessed medically.
- For precautions regarding Cervicalgia, see *Cervical Spondylitis*.
- Liaise with the client's GP if headaches continue after 2 weeks and if the client has not seen their GP.

Heart Attack (Myocardial Infarction)
Heart attacks are caused by damage to the heart muscles resulting from blockage of the coronary arteries. It can cause serious complications including heart failure.

Cautions, Restrictions and Recommendations
- Any treatment should be delayed until recovery and should be given in liaison with client's GP.
- Considerations and cautions are as for *Angina*.

Heart Block
Heart block is an abnormality of the rhythm of the heart. The heart beats at a slower rate and can cause fainting attacks. It can be caused by a congenital abnormality of the conduction of the heart, or due to ischaemic heart disease or infarction. Usually responds to Pacemaker inserted in chest wall instead of using any other form of medical/surgical treatment.

Cautions
See Pacemaker.

Hepatitis
This is an inflammation of the liver caused by viruses, toxic substances or immunological abnormalities. There are three different types of hepatitis:
1. **Hepatitis A** is highly contagious and is transmitted by the faecal–oral route; it is transmitted by ingestion of contaminated food, water or milk. The incubation period is 15–45 days.

2. **Hepatitis B**, also known as serum hepatitis, is more serious than Hepatitis A. It lasts longer and can lead to cirrhosis, cancer of the liver and a carrier state (sufferers can pass it on). It has a long incubation period of up to 2 months and the symptoms may last from weeks to months. The virus is usually transmitted through infected blood, serum or plasma. However, it can also be spread by oral or sexual contact as the virus is present in most body secretions.
3. **Hepatitis C** can cause acute or chronic hepatitis. It can also lead to a carrier state and liver cancer. It is transmitted through blood transfusions or exposure to blood products.

Most clients with Hepatitis are jaundiced, but they can appear to be entirely healthy.
Note: Hepatitis as a side effect of drugs and alcohol intake is *not* infective.

Cautions, Restrictions and Recommendations

- Always consult the GP regarding the infectious state of a client with a history of hepatitis.
- Avoid treatment during acute phases.
- Avoid massage to the abdomen (especially the right upper quadrant) if there is a history of chronic hepatitis (hepatitis lasting for more than 6 months).
- Take special precautions to maintain sterility of equipment and linens.

Hernia

An abnormal protrusion of an organ or part of an organ through the wall of the body cavity in which it normally lies. There are different types of hernia which are given as separate entries below.

Hiatus Hernia

This is the most common type of hernia, when part of the stomach is protruding through the diaphragm into the chest. It may cause no symptoms at all, but can cause acid reflux – acid from stomach passes up the oesophagus causing pain and heartburn.

Cautions, Restrictions and Recommendations

- Avoid positioning clients completely flat on couch; use pillows for comfort and support.
- Discourage bending.
- Encourage eating less.
- Advise on weight reduction and encourage the client to stop smoking.
- Be aware that reflux pain can be similar to Angina.
- Stress reduction can help.

Femoral Hernia

This is a protrusion of the intestine through an abnormal opening at the point at which the femoral artery passes from the abdomen to the thigh.

Cautions, Restrictions and Recommendations

- The client should be advised to consult his or her GP.

- The therapist should avoid undue stretching against resistance and should not massage around the hernia.
- See also *Inginual Hernia*.

KEY NOTE Some types of hernia may require urgent medical attention. See the *Inginual Hernia* entry.

Inginual Hernia

This is a protrusion of the intestine, through an abnormal opening in the groin area.

Cautions, Restrictions and Recommendations

- **Inginual and femoral hernias can become strangulated.**
- **If the hernia is painful and noticeably swollen, and if the patient is constipated or suffers from vomiting, the client should seek medical attention urgently.**

Incisional Hernia

This is the protrusion of intestinal or other tissues through the incision site of a previous surgery.

Cautions, Restrictions and Recommendations

- Avoid increasing intra-abdominal pressure by encouraging the client to raise their head.
- Do not massage the site of the hernia.

Herpes Simplex (Cold Sores)

Herpes Simplex is normally found on the face and around the lips. It begins as an itching sensation, followed by erythema and a group of small blisters. These weep and form crusts. This condition generally persists for approximately 2 or 3 weeks, but may reappear at times of stress or ill health and after exposure to sunlight.

Cautions, Restrictions and Recommendations

- Avoid direct contact with lesions as the condition is highly infectious.
- Advise the client to seek help from their GP or a pharmacist.

Herpes Zoster (Shingles)

This is a painful infection of the sensory nerves by the virus that causes chicken pox. Lesions resemble herpes simplex with erythema and blisters along the lines of the nerves. Areas commonly affected are the back and upper chest wall. The condition is very painful due to acute inflammation of one or more of the peripheral nerves. Severe pain may persist at the site of shingles for months or even years after the apparent healing of the skin.

Cautions, Restrictions and Recommendations

■ Clients should seek help in the acute state from their GP.

■ Massage should be avoided in affected areas because of severe pain and sensitive skin, even after the lesions have healed.

■ This condition is particularly painful on the face and can trigger neuralgia.

■ The condition is not infectious to the therapist.

Hodgkin's Disease

This is a malignant disease of the lymphatic tissues, usually characterised by a painless enlargement of one or more groups of lymph nodes in the neck, armpit, groin, chest, or abdomen. The spleen, liver, bone marrow and bones may also be involved. Apart from the enlarged nodes, there may also be weight loss, fever, profuse sweating at night and itching.

Cautions, Restrictions and Recommendations

■ Clearance from the client's consultant physician is necessary before undertaking any form of treatment.

■ Caution is advised regarding the risk of spreading the disease through the lymphatic system.

■ Clients are vulnerable to infection due to reduced immunity.

■ It is inadvisable to treat if the client is debilitated. However, clients may benefit from a gentle, relaxing treatment.

Hypertension

This is elevation of the arterial blood pressure above the normal range expected in a particular age group. A person is said to be **hypertensive** if the systolic blood pressure is consistently raised above 160 mm Hg and the diastolic is 90 mm Hg or higher.

Complications that may arise from hypertension include ischaemic heart disease, heart failure, kidney failure and cerebral haemorrhage; however, treatment may prevent their development.

Cautions, Restrictions and Recommendations

■ Ensure the client is compliant with their medication.

■ Holistic therapies which produce relaxation can lower blood pressure.

■ Advise the client to reduce their intake of salt and to start a programme of weight reduction, if appropriate.

■ Remember that clients can have hypotension due to their current medication. See *Hypotension*.

■ Oedema of the legs should be reported to the client's GP.

Hypotension

Hypotension is a term given to blood pressure that is lower than normal; a drop of 20 mm Hg systolic pressure and 10 mm Hg diastolic from a person's usual blood pressure results in hypotension. Some people may experience a temporary fall in blood pressure when rising from a horizontal position (known as orthostatic hypotension).

Cautions, Restrictions and Recommendations
- See *Hypertension*; clients can have hypotension as a side effect of their medication for hypertension.
- Care should be taken when clients are sitting or standing up, to avoid falls. Advise gradual movements; first sitting on the edge of the seat or couch to reduce dizziness.
- Liaise with the GP if low blood pressure is suspected as the client may need a change of medication or blood test to exclude anaemia.

Impetigo
This is a superficial but contagious, inflammatory disease caused by streptococcal and staphylococcal bacteria. It is commonly seen on the face and around the ears. Features include weeping blisters which dry to form honey-coloured crusts. (Bacteria are transmitted easily by dirty fingernails and towels.)

Cautions, Restrictions and Recommendations
- As infection can be spread by contact, this condition is contra-indicated to treatment.
- Refer the client to their GP, who will usually prescribe antibiotics to treat the infection.

Irritable Bowel Syndrome
A common condition in which there is recurrent abdominal pain with constipation and/or diarrhoea, and bloating. Clients with stress and hectic lifestyles are more vulnerable to this illness. They usually defecate a few times, usually in the morning, but they may feel that their bowel is not empty, or they may pass pellet-like stools.

Cautions, Restrictions and Recommendations
- Remember that the lower abdomen in particular can be painful and tender.
- Clients with this condition may need easy and quick access to the toilet.
- Advise the client to avoid wind-producing foods, e.g. onions, dry beans.
- Relaxation of any form is helpful.
- Hypnotherapy is confirmed as a useful therapy.

Leukaemia
The term 'leukaemia' refers to any of a group of malignant diseases in which the bone marrow and other blood-forming organs produce an elevated number of certain types of white blood cells. Over-production of these white cells (which are immature or of an abnormal form) suppresses the production of normal white cells, red cells and platelets, leading to an increased susceptibility to infection. Other manifestations or signs include enlargement of the spleen, liver and lymph nodes, spontaneous bruising and anaemia.

Cautions, Restrictions and Recommendations

- Drainage of lymphatics can result in the spread of leukaemia – refer to the GP or consultant for advice.
- Avoid contact with the client if you are suffering from a cold or any other infection.
- Take care when applying pressure in massage to avoid bruising; clients may also have a tendency to bleed.
- The lymph glands, liver and spleen can be very tender.

Lupus Erythematosus

This is a chronic inflammatory disease of the connective tissue, affecting the skin and various internal organs. It is an anto-immune disease and can be diagnosed by the presence of abnormal antibodies in the bloodstream. Typical signs are a red, scaly rash on the face, arthritis and progressive damage to the kidneys. The heart, lungs and brain may also be affected by progressive attacks of inflammation followed by the formation of scar tissue. It can also cause psychiatric illness due to direct brain involvement. In a milder form only the skin is affected.

Cautions, Restrictions and Recommendations

- Care is required when handling as skin lesions might be tender, and joint pain and tenderness may be present.
- Avoid contact if you are suffering from any infectious illness, as the medication for this condition can suppress immunity and patients are prone to infections.

Migraine

This is a specific form of headache, usually unilateral (restricted to one side of the head) and associated with nausea or vomiting and visual disturbances, usually scintillating light waves or zigzags. Clients may experience a visual aura before an attack actually happens. This is usually called a **classical migraine**.

On occasions migraines cause painful, red and watery eyes – **ophthalmoplegic migraine**. Another form of migraine can cause one-sided paralysis, weakness of the face and body. This is called **neuropathic migraine**.

Abdominal migraine can affect children – they present with recurring attacks of abdominal pain with or without nausea and vomiting. Migraine can be treated with simple analgesia or more specialised anti-migraine medication.

Cautions, Restrictions and Recommendations

- Complementary therapies are well known to help migraine sufferers.
- Avoid therapy during acute attacks and especially if you suspect the condition but the client has not received a doctor's diagnosis.
- Remember that stress and tension can increase the frequency and likelihood of attacks.
- Therapies aimed at relaxation can be very helpful.

Remember that women are likely to have more attacks during premenstrual periods, when they are taking contraceptive pills, during the menopause or when starting HRT.

Multiple Sclerosis

This is a disease of the central nervous system, in which the myelin (fatty) sheath covering the nerve fibres is destroyed. Various functions become impaired, including movement and sensations. Multiple sclerosis is characterised by relapses and remissions. It can present with blindness or reduced vision and can lead to severe disability within a short period. In can cause incontinence, loss of balance, tremor and speech problems. Depression and mania can be associated.

Cautions, Restrictions and Recommendations

- Be aware of loss of sensation.
- Be aware that massage and joint movement may trigger muscle spasm.
- Relaxation therapies and exercises may be helpful for decreasing tone in rigid muscles and for preventing stiffness or contractures.
- Temperature extremes may make the symptoms worse.
- Treatments should be slow and gentle and of short duration as clients may tire easily.

Myalgic Encephalomyelitis (Chronic Fatigue Syndrome)

ME is a condition which is characterised by extreme, disabling fatigue that has lasted for at least six months, is made worse by physical or mental exertion and is not resolved by bed rest. The symptom of fatigue is often accompanied by some of the following: muscle pain or weakness, poor co-ordination, joint pain, slight fever, sore throat, painful lymph nodes in the neck and armpits, depression, inability to concentrate and general malaise.

ME can affect people in any age group, but is on the increase in children and adolescents.

Cautions, Restrictions and Recommendations

- This is a condition which can benefit from complementary therapy treatments, but avoid any claim which could be misinterpreted as curative.
- Relaxation can help the client to cope.
- Be aware of tenderness in the muscles and joints.
- Clients may require a lot of support and understanding.

Oedema

Oedema is an abnormal swelling of the body tissues due to an accumulation of tissue fluid. It can be the result of heart failure, liver or kidney disease or chronic varicose veins.

Cautions, Restrictions and Recommendations

- Liaise with the GP regarding the proposed therapy.
- Avoid positioning the client so that they are lying flat if they suffer from shortness of breath.
- Legs can get infected locally if scratched, therefore care is needed.

Osteoporosis

Osteoporosis is characterised by brittle bones, due to ageing and the lack of hormone oestrogen. This affects the body's ability to deposit calcium in the matrix of bone. The disease can also result from prolonged use of steroids. Vulnerability to osteoporosis can be inherited. Bones can break easily and vertebrae can collapse.

Cautions, Restrictions and Recommendations

■ Avoid vigorous movements as there is a chance of spontaneous fractures.
■ Take care when handling clients as they may have tender bones.
■ Be aware of causing vertebral damage. Take care to make clients comfortable and avoid any movement that may cause pain.

Pacemaker

A pacemaker is an artificial electronic device implanted under the skin. It stimulates and controls the heart rate by sending electrical stimuli to the heart. It is usually installed for heart block (a very slow heart beat) and placed to one side of the upper chest.

Cautions, Restrictions and Recommendations

■ The site of pacemaker is likely to be tender, so avoid it.
■ Be aware that clients are likely to be on other medication.
■ Seek GP approval before offering treatment.

Parkinson's Disease

Parkinson's disease causes damage to the grey matter of brain, known as basal ganglia. This causes involuntary tremors of limbs, with stiffness, rigidity and a shuffling gait. The face lacks expression and movements are slow. Patients may suffer from depression, confusion and anxiety. Therapists should be aware that, since Parkinson's disease is a degenerative condition, symptoms may begin slowly and the disease progresses at different rates in different individuals.

Cautions, Restrictions and Recommendations

■ Clients are likely to be depressed and, as with many conditions, a sympathetic ear may be beneficial.
■ Sufferers are slow and, therefore, need time to move, speak and express themselves.
■ Falls can happen easily, therefore, take special care when clients stand up or change direction when walking.
■ Medication may cause hypotension – see *Hypotension*.
■ Prepare additional tissue papers in case of excessive salivation.
■ Gentle, slow, relaxation treatments of short duration are usually beneficial.

Phlebitis

This is an inflammation of the wall of a vein, most commonly seen in the legs as a complication of varicose veins. A segment of the vein becomes tender and painful; the surrounding skin may feel hot and appear red. Thrombosis may develop as a result of phlebitis (thrombophlebitis) with subsequent DVT (Deep Vein Thrombosis). DVT can cause clots in the lungs (or other organs) with serious consequences.

Cautions, Restrictions and Recommendations

- The site of phlebitis can be tender and, therefore, careful handling is essential.
- Massage is to be avoided to prevent dislodging of clots.
- Liaise with the GP if DVT is suspected.
- Remember that clots, particularly from the legs can travel to the organs, e.g. lungs causing pulmonary embolism.
- Medication can include warfarin to prevent blood clotting. Patients can bruise easily and, therefore, special care is needed.
- See *Thrombosis* and *Pulmonary Embolism*.

Psoriasis

This is a chronic, inflammatory skin condition. Psoriasis results in the development of well-defined red plaques, varying in size and shape and covered by white or silvery scales. Any area of the body may be affected by psoriasis but the most commonly affected sites are the face, elbows, knees, nails, chest and abdomen (it can also affect joints). Psoriasis may occur on the scalp. Psoriasis is aggravated by stress and trauma but is improved by exposure to sunlight.

Cautions, Restrictions and Recommendations

- Caution is advised regarding the application of oils.
- Acute flare-up of psoriasis can cause painful and tender skin lesions and care is needed during massage.
- Stress-relieving therapies may be beneficial.

Pulmonary Embolism

This occurs when a blood clot is carried into the lungs, where it blocks the flow of blood to the pulmonary tissue. This is a very serious condition and can be life threatening. Clients who suffer from this condition may require hospitalisation and medication to thin the blood, e.g. warfarin. This condition presents with chest pain, a cough and shortness of breath.

Cautions, Restrictions and Recommendations

- Any form of holistic therapy is to be avoided during an acute attack and advice should be sought from the client's GP before offering treatment.

Raynaud's Syndrome

This is a disorder of the peripheral arterioles, characterised by spasm in the vascular smooth muscle of the fingers and toes. It is generally brought on by cold or emotional upset. The effect is a pallor or discoloration of the skin, due to the presence of poorly oxygenated haemoglobin. The extremities can become painful and uncomfortable, and this is usually followed by redness and stiffness of the toes and fingers.

Cautions, Restrictions and Recommendations

- Stress-relieving therapies may be beneficial; reducing stress can help to decrease sympathetic stimulation, so relaxing the smooth muscle of the blood vessels.
- Massage may help to improve stiffness of joints and will increase local circulation.
- Use of heat or cold packs are contra-indicated.
- Clients with this condition may require medical treatment and it is important to liaise with the GP.

Ringworm

Ringworm is a fungal infection of the skin, which begins as small red papules that gradually increase in size to form a ring. Affected areas vary in severity from mild scaling to inflamed itchy areas.

Cautions, Restrictions and Recommendations

- This condition is infectious and, therefore, contact therapy is better avoided until the condition has cleared.
- Advise the client to consult their GP.

Scabies

This is a contagious, parasitic skin condition, caused by a female mite. The mite burrows into the horny layer of the skin where she lays her eggs. The first noticeable symptom of this condition is severe itching which worsens at night; papules, pustules and crusted lesions may also develop.

Common sites for this infestation are the ulnar borders of the hand, palms of the hands and between the fingers and toes. Other sites include the axillary folds, buttocks, breasts in the female and external genitalia in the male.

Cautions, Restrictions and Recommendations

- This condition is infectious and, therefore, contact therapy is better avoided until the condition has cleared.
- Advise the client to seek medical help.

Stroke

A stroke is the result of a block in the blood flow to the brain, caused by an embolus in a cerebral blood vessel. This may bring about a sudden attack of weakness, affecting one side of the body, due to the interruption to the flow of blood to the brain. Strokes can vary in severity from a passing weakness or tingling in a limb, to a profound paralysis and coma.

Sometimes the term is used to describe **cerebral haemorrhage** in which an artery or congenital cyst of blood vessels in the brain burst, resulting in damage to the brain. This causes similar signs to thrombus of cerebral vessels. Haemorrhage is usually associated with severe headaches and can cause neck stiffness.

Cautions, Restrictions and Recommendations

- Therapists normally deal with clients who are recovered or who are recovering from a stroke and relaxation therapies can benefit and aid recovery.
- Be aware of muscle spasm and jerking movements in a paralysed limb.
- Clients may need help onto and off the couch.
- Neck massage is best avoided.

Thrombosis

This is a condition in which the blood changes from a liquid to a solid state and produces a blood clot. Thrombosis in the wall of an artery obstructs the blood flow to the tissue it supplies; in the brain this is one cause of a stroke and in the heart it results in a heart attack (coronary thrombosis). Thrombosis may also occur in a vein (Deep Vein Thrombosis – DVT) such as in the leg. The thrombus (blood clot) may be detached from its site of formation and be carried in the blood to lodge in another part.

Cautions, Restrictions and Recommendations

- See *Pulmonary Embolism.*

Rosacea

This is a chronic, inflammatory disease of the face in which the skin appears abnormally red. The condition is gradual and begins with flushing of the checks and nose. As the condition progresses it may become pustular. Aggravating factors include heat, spicy foods, hot drinks, alcohol, the menopause, the elements and stress.

Cautions, Restrictions and Recommendations

- Stress reduction can help.
- Specialised oils may help, but care must be taken due to the sensitivity of the skin.
- Avoid over stimulation of the skin as this may aggravate the condition.
- Encourage a reduction in alcohol intake and avoidance of hot, spicy foods.

Sciatica

This is lower back pain which can affect the buttock and thigh. On occasions it radiates to the leg and foot. It can, in severe cases, cause numbness and weakness of the lower limb. It can result from a prolapse of the discs between the spinal vertebrae, a tumour or a blood clot (thrombosis). Diabetes or heavy alcohol intake can produce symptoms of sciatica. This condition tends to recur and may require strong analgesia or surgery in severe cases.

Cautions, Restrictions and Recommendations

- Avoid unnecessary manipulation.
- Check the couch for comfort.
- Be aware that climbing on to or lying on the couch can produce pain.
- Relaxation and massage can be helpful and the aim in treatments should be to relax muscles and prevent spasms.
- Liaise with the GP regarding diagnosis and the possible benefit from physiotherapy.

Thyroid Disease

The thyroid gland is an endocrine organ which secretes **thyroxine**, a hormone essential for metabolism and body functions. Patients can present with an enlarged gland at the lower end of the neck (goitre). On occasions this may be malignant and surgery or radiation may be required. There are two types of thyroid problem:

1. **Hyperthyroidism** – overproduction of thyroxine may present with anxiety, tremors, palpitations, overeating, diarrhoea and loss of weight. Treatment is with iodine, carbimazole, or surgery may be needed.
2. **Hypothyroidism** – this is caused by an under-active thyroid. The amount of thyroxine hormone produced is not sufficient. Clients may present with dry skin, coarse and dry hair, loss of hair, weight gain, abnormal periods in women, a puffy face and cold intolerance. Hypothyroidism may be caused by inflammatory disease or following hyperthyroid treatment. Clients with this condition need hormone replacement with thyroxine tablets.

Cautions, Restrictions and Recommendations

- Liaise with the GP to maintain compliance with taking medication.
- Avoid massage of the lower neck if there is thyroid enlargement or a sensitive operation site.
- Remember that clients with hyperthyroidism are intolerant of heat and those with hypothyroidism are intolerant of cold.

Tinea Pedis (Athletes Foot)

This is a highly contagious condition which is easily transmitted in damp, moist conditions such as swimming pools, saunas and showers. Athletes foot appears as flaking skin between the toes which then becomes soft and soggy. The skin may also split and the soles of the feet may occasionally be affected.

Cautions, Restrictions and Recommendations

- See *Ringworm*.

Ulcers

An ulcer is a break in the skin or a break in the lining of the alimentary tract that fails to heal and is accompanied by inflammation. **Peptic**, **duodenal** and **gastric ulcers** can present with increased acidity, epigastric pain (in the middle of the upper abdomen) and heartburn. This may be worse when hungry or after consumption of irritating foods and alcohol, e.g. spicy and fatty foods, mayonnaise, wines and spirits. It can present with symptoms similar to those of a hiatus hernia, and reflux.

Cautions, Restrictions and Recommendations

- Remember that peptic, gastric and duodenal ulcers may be suspected when epigastric pain, heartburn and/or acidity are present, but a definite diagnosis is only made after full investigation. Encourage the client to see their GP.

- Encourage small meals, avoidance of acidic food and fatty meals.
- Relaxation can help reduce the stress which can provoke ulcer pain.
- Massage can cause stomach pain if performed deeply.
- It is preferable to perform therapy at least an hour after meals, but avoid treatment when the client has an empty stomach.

Varicose Veins and Ulcers

Twisted and enlarged veins usually appear on the surface of lower limbs but can present in men as piles in the scrotum, or at the lower end of the oesophagus. Varicose veins have defective valves which means that the blood stagnates causing pain, oedema or possibly thrombosis. The tissue of the lower legs can become thin and unhealthy, causing an ulcer. Ulcers can also develop after a superficial injury. The injury does not heal due to the poor circulation caused by reduced venous return.

Cautions, Restrictions and Recommendations

- See *Phlebitis, Oedema* and *Thrombosis*.
- Liaise with the GP.
- Avoid direct pressure to affected areas.
- Avoid any infected areas.
- Encourage foot elevation.

Whiplash

This is a condition produced by damage to the muscles, ligaments, intervertebral discs or nerve tissues of the cervical region by sudden hyperextension and/or flexion of the neck. The most common cause is a road traffic accident when acceleration or deceleration causes a sudden stretch of the tissue around the cervical spine. It may also occur as a result of hard impact sports. Whiplash can present with pain, limitation of neck movements with muscle tenderness. This can start hours to days after the accident, and it may take months to recover. This is usually associated with complicated physical, psychological and legal issues.

Cautions, Restrictions and Recommendations

- The condition may last for a few months or years.
- Clients may be involved in legal cases. It is best, therefore, to avoid making any comments about reasons for the condition, the prognosis or the suitability of a particular therapy.
- Bear in mind that, if seeking compensation, the client may have an interest in delaying healing.
- Ascertain that the client is not seeking a cure; ensure that you offer no promise of a cure either.
- Take care when massaging the neck and avoid manipulation or moving vigorously.
- Relaxation exercises can help.
- Holistic therapies may help clients to cope with their condition.

CHAPTER 4

Understanding imbalance

Any form of therapeutic bodywork, whether massage or healing, is based on the principles that our bodies are electromagnetic and energetic in nature, and if this energy is influenced positively, it can help to promote balance and a sense of well-being.

In order to understand how emotions can cause energy blocks in the tissues of our body, it is useful to have an insight into the oriental systems of body circuits called **meridians** and the subtle energy fields of **chakras**. If energy is not flowing freely, our bodies are not working to their optimum level and this can result in physical and emotional imbalance.

The aim of this chapter is to explore the concept of **yin and yang** from Chinese medicine, the role of meridians in physical and emotional balance (page 44) and the role of the chakras in subtle energy therapy (page 67).

YIN AND YANG

In order to understand the role of meridians, first it is important to examine the oriental concept of yin and yang. This is the philosophy that forms the foundation of Chinese medicine.

Yin and yang represent a duality of oneness. It is a way of expressing opposite and complementary states of energy such as night and day, winter and summer, hot and cold, male and female.

Figure 4.1 The symbol for yin and yang

The term yin is applied to characteristics that are cool, wet, passive, introverted, and female; yang is a general term used to describe characteristics that are hot, dry, active, extroverted and male.

It is important to understand that the terms used to describe yin and yang are *relative* rather than absolute states. There is nothing that is purely yin or purely yang; each contains a part of the other in order to represent wholeness.

Everybody, despite their gender, possesses varying degrees of yin and yang characteristics. The subtle balance is constantly changing and, in the same way, every aspect of the universe changes. There are cycles of light and seasons, which reflect the constant shift between the polar opposites.

Understanding the energetic roles of yin and yang is the key to any therapeutic application.

> **KEY NOTE** The primary function of yin is to cool, moisten, relax and promote sleep. The primary function of yang is to warm, energise and stimulate.

When yin and yang are balanced within your life, you experience health. When they are imbalanced, ill health can arise. If a person's yin energy is deficient, the symptoms are likely to be a feeling of heat, thirst and restlessness. If a person's yang energy is deficient they are likely to feel chilly, tired and unmotivated.

A person's condition, whether excessively yin or yang, will have a direct impact on how the energy flows in the meridians. An excessively cold condition may restrict the flow of energy along a meridian, while too much heat may cause an excess of energy to flow along a meridian.

The concept of yin and yang may be used as a guide when helping clients to restore balance and overall health. The application of this ancient theory is discussed below.

The Application of Yin and Yang

Yin and yang can be defined with reference to the **eight principles of change**:

Yin	**Yang**
■ cold	■ hot
■ empty	■ full
■ deep	■ surface
■ imbalanced towards the yin	■ imbalanced towards the yang

To illustrate this in simple terms, if a person is feeling chilly and lacking in energy, they will be imbalanced towards the yin. The condition is likely to be longer-term and chronic. If a person has a fever and a full feeling in the chest, the condition is imbalanced towards the yang. The symptoms are likely to be short-term and acute.

These are extreme examples of excessive yin and yang states. However, in practice most people are likely to suffer from combinations of yin and yang conditions.

For example, when touching a client's back, you find the upper back to be hot (yang) and the lower back to be cool (yin). Relating this to the eight principles of change, the upper back would be considered full (yang) with the tension being very much on the surface. The lower back would be considered empty (yin) with the tension being so deep that it has a hollow or empty feeling.

In order to restore health, we need to balance the opposing extremes. In other words, the extreme yang part must relax and become more supple (or more yin) and the extreme yin must become more active, vital and full (or more yang).

> *KEY NOTE* With any form of bodywork, it is important to understand that we are not only dealing with surface tension, but also with the underlying organs and the meridians that supply these organs with energy. Problems arising with organs, nerves, muscles and meridians are all connected. We should never forget the whole, as one problem may affect the body in the form of a compensatory imbalance elsewhere.

Having a deeper understanding of meridians can help us to recognise that problems in a certain part of the body correspond to problems in specific organs. We can work on these areas in order to address the imbalance.

MERIDIANS

The human body is a natural energy source which generates electrical energy within the ionic environment of the cells and tissues. Body fluids contain electrically-charged ions which can cause a current to flow. Body meridians are thought to contain a colourless, free-flowing, non-cellular fluid, which conveys this electrical energy throughout the body.

Although the meridians are categorised in terms of the organs and tissues that they supply, they are thought to form a single continuous circuit which conveys electromagnetic energy throughout the body.

The body's circuit of electrical energy is divided into 14 major meridians; there are 12 organic meridians and two storage meridians. Body meridians are named according to the internal structures they supply. Each of the organic meridians supply a group of muscles in the body, as well as a group of internal tissues.

Organic Meridians
Yin Meridians

Six of the organic meridians are called yin meridians. The yin circuit conveys negative electromagnetic energy throughout the body and supplies the yin organs:

- heart
- lungs
- liver
- spleen
- kidney
- pericardium.

The yin meridians have a common purpose which is to alter, circulate and store blood and energy (chi). They are located deep in the body.

Yang Meridians

The remaining six organic circuits are called yang meridians. The yang meridians convey positive electromagnetic energy throughout the body and supply the yang organs:

- stomach
- small intestine
- large intestine
- gall bladder
- urinary bladder
- triple warmer (the three zones of energy in the torso).

The yang meridians are closer to the surface and are all part of the digestive system.

It is important to understand that no organ operates independently within the meridian network. Each yin organ and its meridian, works in line with a corresponding organ and meridian. So, the meridians function in pairs, each one being made up of one yin meridian and one yang meridian. Energy or chi, moves from the head towards the feet through the yang meridians on the back of the body and from the feet to the head through the yin meridians on the front.

The Storage Meridians

The storage meridians (the **conception vessel** and the **governing vessel**) both help to create balance among the 12 organic meridians by dispersing excess chi to deficient meridians. They also help to unite the organic meridians by allowing chi flow to adjust when there is a blockage.

> **KEY NOTE** When working along a specific meridian, remember that you are also working on a related organ. When pressing on a point along a meridian, energy is boosted along the pathway to the corresponding organ.

Yin, Yang and Emotional State

It is important to realise that emotions can upset the natural balance and flow of electromagnetic energy in the body, by subtly altering the chemical state of the body's tissues and their ionic conductivity. Yin emotions such as depression, fear, disappointment, grief, withdrawal and shame can cause the body's tissues to be flooded with negative electromagnetic energy. The negative energy that permeates the body's system then causes negative congestion. This deprives the yang circuit and the corresponding muscles and tissues of positive energy.

Conversely, an excess of yang emotions such as anger, agitation, impatience, frustration, jealousy, hostility, envy and defensiveness can flood the tissues with positive electromagnetic energy. This depletes the yin circuits along with the muscles and tissues supplied by them.

The Heart Meridian

The heart meridian begins at the heart and surfaces in the centre of the axilla. The meridian passes down the inside of the arm, crosses the inner point of the elbow fold, and runs through to the tip of the little finger.

Common Symptoms of Imbalance

PHYSICAL	EMOTIONAL
hot or cold hands and feet	excessive laughter
red complexion	hysteria
nervousness	lack of joy
irritability	expressionless appearance
mental or emotional disturbance	
insomnia, disturbed sleep or excessive dreaming	
cardiovascular disorders	
brain or nervous system disorders	
speech problems	
spontaneous sweating	
poor memory of important life events	

KEY NOTE The heart meridian is the centre of emotional and mental consciousness. It is associated with passion, mental clarity and joy.

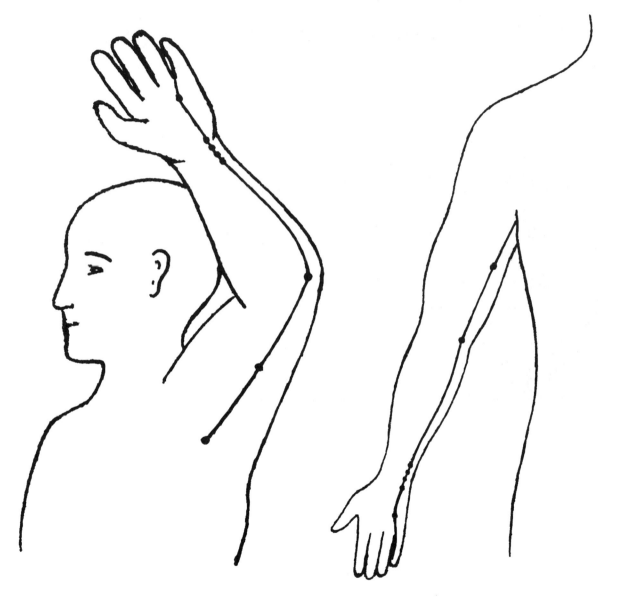

Figure 4.2 The heart meridian

The Lung Meridian

The lung meridian runs from deep in the body within the lung to surface in the hollow area by the front shoulder. It then passes over the shoulder and down the front of the arm, running along the biceps muscle. It goes down the arm to the wrist just below the base of the thumb and ends at the thumbnail.

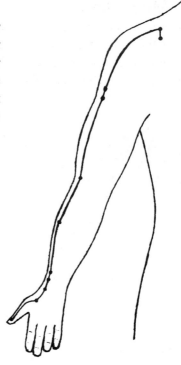

Figure 4.3 The lung meridian

Common Symptoms of Imbalance

PHYSICAL	EMOTIONAL
asthma	chronic or long-term grief, sorrow
bronchitis	claustrophobia
congestion in the chest	compulsive behaviour
coughing	restlessness
breathing difficulties	
pneumonia	
excessive mucus	
sore throat	
loss of voice	
deficient or excessive perspiration	
collapsed or hollow chest	

KEY NOTE In Chinese medicine, the lungs are the rulers of energy. How deeply we breathe shapes the energy and gives it its definition to provide the quality and quantity of energy required for respiration.

The Liver Meridian

The liver meridian begins at a point inside the big toenail, passes over the top of the foot, continues above the inside of the ankle, runs past the inside of the knee and along the inner thigh. It proceeds through the genital region, upwards to the sides of the body and then ends at the ribs just over the liver (for the meridian on the right side of the body) and just over the spleen (on the left side).

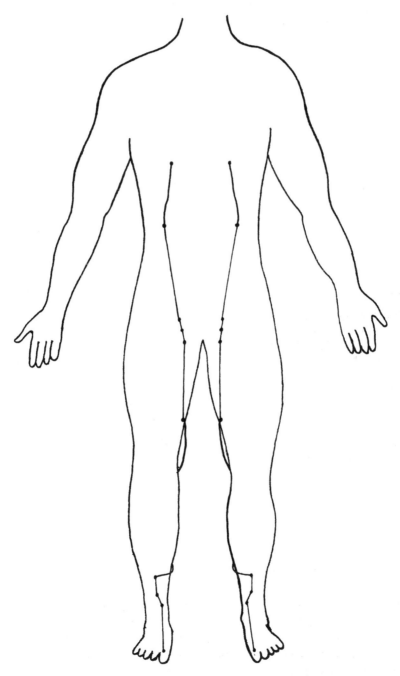

Figure 4.4 The liver meridian

Common Symptoms of Imbalance

PHYSICAL	EMOTIONAL
red face	anger
pale, drawn face	frustration
headaches (at the top of the head)	depression
migraines	lack of will
dizziness	
pain and swelling in the genitals	
menstrual pain, irregular periods, premenstrual syndrome	
disorders of the eye and vision	
muscle spasms, seizures, convulsions	
pale fingernails, ridges in nails, cracked nails	
pain relating to tendons	
allergies	
easily bruised	
dandruff and hair loss	

KEY NOTE In Chinese medicine, the liver and liver meridian are considered to control the life force. The liver meridian is associated with expression of the will and with creativity – when life energy is weak it is usually indicative of a troubled liver.

The Spleen Meridian

The spleen meridian begins at the inside of the big toe at the nail and then runs along the inside of the foot, it turns upward in front of the ankle bone, then ascends along the inside of the calf to the knee. From there, the meridian runs up through the genital region, through the abdomen, proceeds to the spleen itself, and then to the stomach. The meridian continues upwards, along the side of the body and chest area to the outside of the breast.

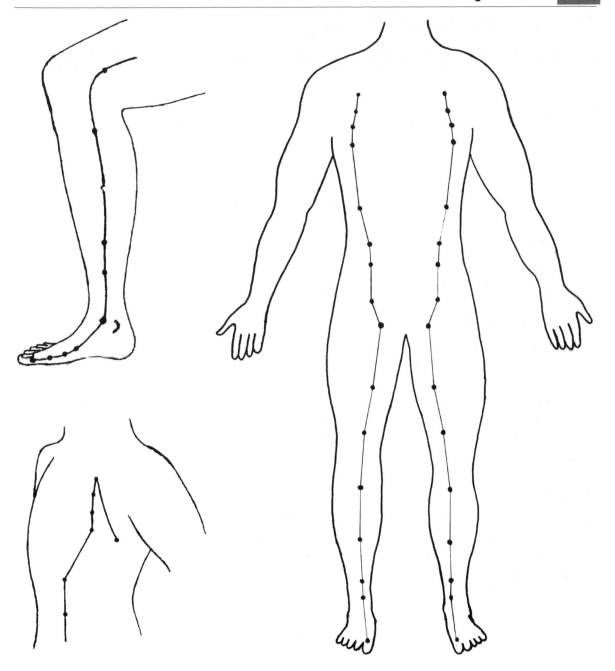

Figure 4.5 The spleen meridian

Common Symptoms of Imbalance

PHYSICAL	EMOTIONAL
digestive problems – dyspepsia, constipation and diarrhoea	excessive worry
heartburn, acid indigestion	sensitivity
nausea	obsession
belching and gas	lack of awareness
immune deficiency or disorders	
lymphatic problems (swollen lymph nodes)	
abdominal distension	
appetite imbalance	
hypoglycaemia or diabetes	
heavy, aching body	
knee or thigh problems	
memory problems	
vomiting after eating	

KEY NOTE In Chinese medicine, the spleen is regarded as the primary organ of digestion, passing chi to the small and large intestines. When the spleen is weakened by excessive consumption of sugar and acidic foods, it is unable to pass sufficient energy to the intestine. This often results in chronic indigestion and constipation.

The Kidney Meridian

The kidney meridian starts at the little toe and crosses under the foot to the inner edge of the instep. It circles the anklebone towards the heel, then rises along the inside of the calf to the inner thigh. At the pubic region it goes external for a short distance and re-emerges over the abdomen and chest extending to the clavicle.

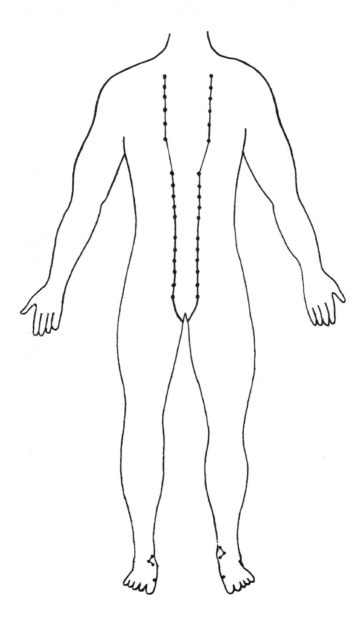

Figure 4.6 The kidney meridian

Common Symptoms of Imbalance

PHYSICAL	EMOTIONAL
cold extremities (especially the feet)	fearful, easily frightened
achy or weak bones	chronic anxiety
darkness under the eyes	foolhardiness
drowsiness, lack of energy	
diarrhoea	
dizziness on standing	
tinnitus	
oedema	
hearing loss	
low back pain	
irregular menstruation	
premenstrual syndrome	
reproductive problems	
painful or hot soles of feet	
urinary incontinence	
sexual problems	
hypertension	
hair loss	

KEY NOTE In Chinese medicine, the kidneys are responsible for strength and constitutional vitality of the body. They control the essential energy within each cell of the body and thereby maintain the health, vitality and function of every organ, system and sense.

The Circulation or Pericardium Meridian

The circulation or pericardium meridian starts internally at the surface of the heart and emerges just outside each nipple. It follows around the axilla and travels down the inside of the arm to the wrist ending at the thumb-side corner of the middle fingernail.

Common Symptoms of Imbalance

PHYSICAL	EMOTIONAL
stiffness of spasm in the arm and elbow	timidity
distended chest and ribs	anxiety
discomfort in chest	nervousness
hot palms	insensitivity
red face	rude behaviour
sexual dysfunction	excessive laughter
painful or swollen underarm area	
tension in upper chest	
painful, stiff head and neck	

KEY NOTE The circulation or pericardium meridian does not correspond directly to an organ.

The Stomach Meridian

The stomach meridian starts below the eyes, descends to the sides of the mouth and the jaw, from where a branch rises to the forehead. It also continues along the side of the throat to the collarbone and over the chest and abdomen to the pubic area. From there, it passes along the front of the thigh to the outside of the kneecap. Below the kneecap, the meridian divides into two branches, one that ends at the second toe and one that ends at the third toe.

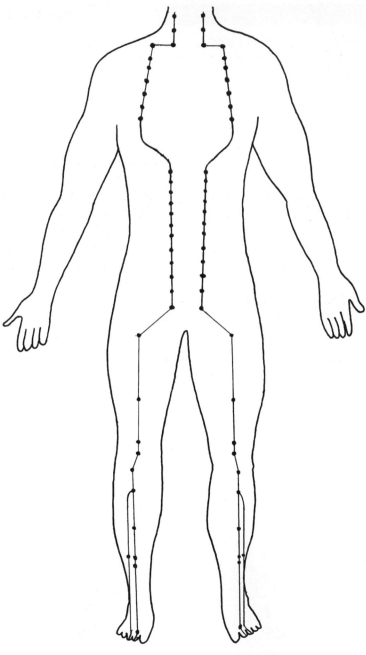

Figure 4.7 The stomach meridian

Common Symptoms of Imbalance

PHYSICAL	EMOTIONAL
distension of the upper abdomen	critical
abdominal pain	lack of understanding
jaw tension	lack of compassion
knee pain	anxiety and nervous tension
lip or mouth sores	emotionally unstable
vomiting	
frequent hunger or thirst	
neck or throat swelling	
yawning	
groaning	

KEY NOTE In Chinese medicine, the stomach and spleen are considered to be connected, one providing energy to the other. As the stomach meridian begins at the mouth, it is said to govern the mouth, tongue and oesophagus, thereby controlling the preparation of food for digestion.

The Small Intestine Meridian

The small intestine meridian begins at the outside of the nail on the little finger, trails the back of the hand to the wrist and flows from the outside of the ulna to the elbow. It follows the back of the arm up to the shoulder joint, where it crosses the scapula to the clavicle. From here, the meridian continues up the side of the neck and over the cheek to the ear.

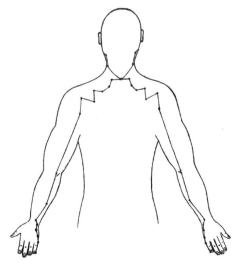

Figure 4.8 The small intestine meridian

Common Symptoms of Imbalance

PHYSICAL	EMOTIONAL
distension of the lower abdomen	lack of mental clarity (deficient chi)
arm pain	lack of joy (deficient chi)
shoulder pain and tension	over emotional (excess chi)
swollen cheeks	hysteria (excess chi)
difficulty in turning head to one side	
sore or stiff elbow joint	
eye soreness or redness	
disorders relating to the small intestine	

KEY NOTE In Chinese medicine, imbalances in the small intestine prevent the smooth transfer of energy from the food to the stomach, resulting in digestive disorders. The small intestine is considered to be linked with the heart, helping to bring clarity of mind.

The Large Intestine Meridian

The large intestine meridian starts at the index finger on the outside of the nail (towards the thumb), runs through the crease between the thumb and the index finger, then passes up the thumb-side edge of the arm to the edge of the shoulder. It then crosses the shoulder and neck to the cheek, touches the upper lip and ends at the nostril.

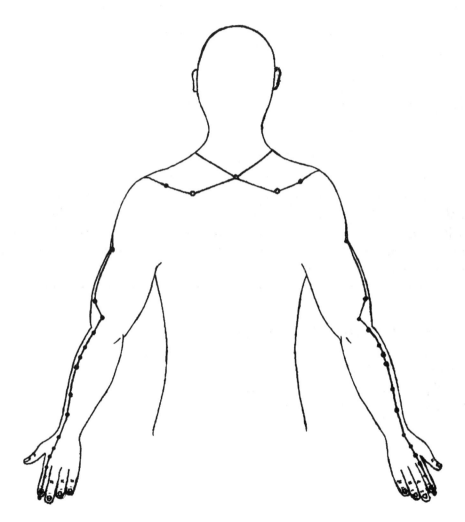

Figure 4.9 The large intestine meridian

Common Symptoms of Imbalance

PHYSICAL	EMOTIONAL
constipation	excessive worry
diarrhoea	grief and sadness
headache	compulsive attention to detail
shoulder pain	stubbornness
nasal congestion	
toothache	

KEY NOTE In Chinese medicine the large intestine is considered to perform the function of elimination, both in a physical and metaphysical sense. That is, the condition of the large intestine reflects the mind and body's capacity to eliminate those experiences, beliefs and emotions we no longer need. This enables us to grow as individuals. The large intestine is also responsible for sending energy downwards into the body and, thus, grounds us to the earth.

The Gall Bladder Meridian

The first thing to notice about the gall bladder meridian is that it zigzags back and forth over the head and that it zigzags down both sides of the body. Secondly, it is one of the longest meridians. The meridian begins at the outside corner of each eye, loops around the ear to the neck, goes back over the head to the forehead above the eyes, then over the head again to the back of the neck. From there it drops down the neck and over the front of each shoulder. It then zigzags down the sides of the body, along the outside of each leg, over the front of the ankles, and ends at the fourth toe.

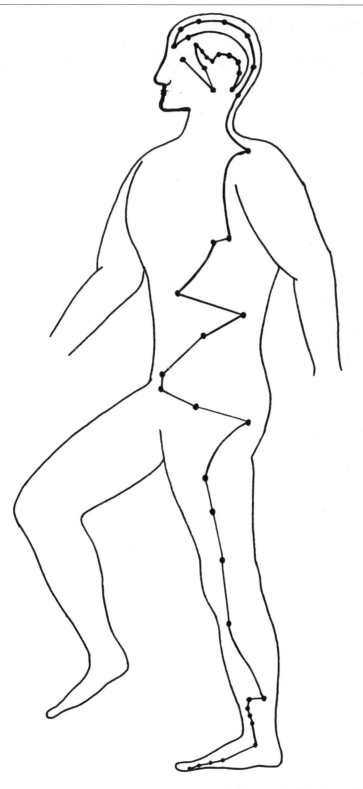

Figure 4.10 The gall bladder meridian

Common Symptoms of Imbalance

PHYSICAL	EMOTIONAL
headache (temple) and migraine	anger and frustration (excess chi)
eye and ear pain	depression and lack of will (deficient chi)
joint stiffness and pain	
tightness and pain in the sides of the chest	
nausea and vomiting	
yellow colour in eyes	
stiffness in fourth toe	
gall stones	

KEY NOTE In Chinese medicine, the gall bladder is seen as an external manifestation of the liver energy. Therefore, liver symptoms become more pronounced when the gall bladder is imbalanced. The Chinese say that when the gall bladder is balanced, good judgement and clear thinking is made possible; when the organ is unbalanced frustration and clouded judgement will result.

The Bladder Meridian

The bladder meridian begins at the inside corner of the eye, passes over the forehead and the top of the head, then continues down the back in four lines, two on either side of the spine. The four lines continue over the buttocks and down the legs, where two meet behind each knee. A single line then passes down each leg along the centre line of the calf behind the outer ankle, and ends at the outer tip of the little toe.

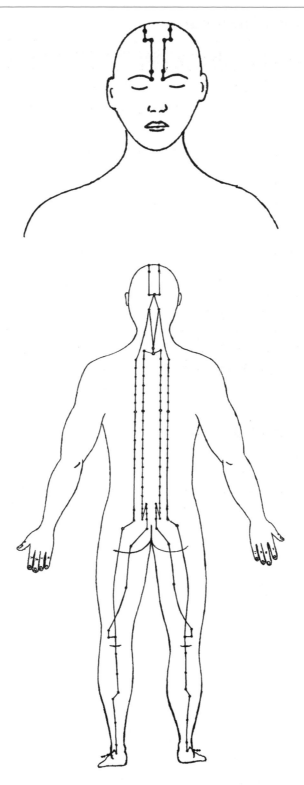

Figure 4.11 The bladder meridian

Common Symptoms of Imbalance

PHYSICAL	EMOTIONAL
back problems	paranoia
bladder infections jealousy	
incontinence	excessive suspicion
hip or sacrum problems fear	
pain on inside corner of eye	chronic anxiety
rounded shoulders	
spasm or pain at back of calf	
stiffness in little toe	
aching feet after standing	

KEY NOTE In Chinese medicine, the bladder is part of the system that includes the kidneys and the reproductive organs. By boosting energy along the bladder meridian, you strengthen not only the bladder itself but every organ in the body.

The Triple Warmer Meridian

The triple warmer meridian begins on the outside corner of the nail on the fourth finger and runs up the middle of the outside of the arm to the top of the shoulder. It continues over the shoulder to the clavicle, up the back of the neck and circles around the back of the ear. It then continues to the outer corner of the eyebrow.

Common Symptoms of Imbalance

PHYSICAL	EMOTIONAL
distended abdomen	none
colds and fevers	
deafness	
pain behind ear	
elbow problems	
swollen jaw	
slow metabolism, overweight	
fast metabolism, hyperactive	

KEY NOTE In Chinese medicine the triple warmer, also known as the triple heater meridian, does not relate to a specific organ, but is believed to control fluids within the body, specifically water and the endocrine system. The triple warmer receives its name from the three centres of activity within the body that, as they function, create heat:
- the upper warmer is associated with the heart and the lungs
- the middle warmer is associated with the liver, spleen and stomach
- the lower warmer with the kidneys, bladder, small and large intestines.

The Conception Vessel Meridian

The conception vessel meridian starts in the pelvic cavity, drops down and emerges in the perineum, just between the anus and the genitals. It then crosses through the genital area to the top of the pubic bone, runs up the midline of the abdomen, chest and neck and ends just below the lower lip.

Common Symptoms of Imbalance

PHYSICAL	EMOTIONAL
asthma	none
coughing	
epilepsy	
eczema	
hay fever	
head and neck pain	
laryngitis	
lung problems	
mouth sores	
pneumonia	
genital disorders	
itching	
painful abdominal skin	

KEY NOTE In Chinese medicine, the conception vessel is seen as the regulator of the peripheral nervous system and, along with the governing vessel (see below), it controls the other 12 meridians. It creates balance by uniting the organ meridians, allowing energy flow to adjust when there is a blockage. In addition to providing energy to all of the peripheral nerves, the conception vessel also governs menstruation and the development of the foetus in women.

The Governing Vessel Meridian

The governing vessel meridian begins in the pelvic cavity and then drops down and emerges below the genital area. It then passes to the tip of the coccyx. From her, it moves upward across the sacrum and along the spine, up over the head towards the upper lip. It then goes under the lip to the upper gum.

Common Symptoms of Imbalance

PHYSICAL	EMOTIONAL
headaches and pain in the eyes	none
stiffness in the spine	
back pain or tension	
dizziness	
eye problems	
cold extremities	
fevers	
haemorrhoids	
insomnia	
neck pain	
spinal problems	
rounded shoulders, heavy head	

KEY NOTE In Chinese medicine, the governing vessel is the regulator of the nervous system and, along with the conception vessel, it controls the other 12 meridians. Like the conception vessel, it allows excess energy to pass through it to other meridians that may be deficient in energy. The Chinese think of this as an 'extra meridian'.

CHAKRAS

Everything that happens to us on an emotional level has an energetic impact on the **subtle body** (or **aura**), which in turn has an impact on the physical body. Chakras are thought to be non-physical energy centres located about an inch away from the physical body. The energy field of each chakra extends beyond the visible body of matter in the subtle body.

It is important to remember that chakras do not have a physical form and any illustration of the chakras is merely a visual aid to the imagination and not a literal, physical reality.

Chakras are a way of describing the flow of subtle energy and are said each to be related to an endocrine gland, which the chakra is thought to influence. The chakras exist in a state of synchrony and balance. However, with stress, the chakras can lose their ability to synchronise and they become unbalanced.

If negative energy accumulates in a chakra, the function of the chakra becomes impaired. Ultimately, this can lead to energy blocks. If one chakra ceases to function, this creates an imbalance as the other chakras attempt to compensate, creating additional strain on the energy system.

An accumulation of negative energy in one or more chakras can manifest itself as an emotional or physical condition. Often we are only aware of a change in the physical body as our attention is drawn to pain or disease; we do not usually link the symptom to a cause within the subtle body.

So chakras are the focal points for the subtle energies and are the key to restoring balancing. By placing hands along the axis of the chakras, energy can be aligned and harmony restored. By working with the subtle energy, the chakras may be strengthened and energy may be increased, decreased or balanced as required by the body at the time of the treatment.

The Base or Root Chakra

Location	at the base of the spine
Relevance	the foundation chakra; linked with nature and planet Earth; concerned with all issues of a physical nature – the body, the senses, sensuality, a person's sex, survival, aggression and self-defence; at a physical level, it is linked to the endocrine system through the adrenal glands; its energies also affect the lower parts of the pelvis, the hips, legs and feet
Imbalance	if this chakra is unbalanced it can make a person feel as if they are ungrounded and unfocused; they may feel weak, lack confidence and be unable to achieve their goals
Colour association	red

The Sacral Chakra

Location	at the level of the sacrum between the naval and the base chakra
Relevance	concerned with all issues of creativity and sexuality; at the physical level, it is linked to the testes in the male and the ovaries in the female; its energies also affect the urino-genital organs, the uterus, the kidneys, the lower digestive organs and the lower back
Imbalance	a person with an imbalance in this chakra may bury their emotions and be overly sensitive; an imbalance may also lead to sexual difficulties and energy blocks which affect creativity
Colour association	orange

The Solar Plexus Chakra

Location	at approximately waist level
Relevance	relates to our emotions, self-esteem and self-worth; feelings such as fear, anxiety, insecurity, jealousy and anger are generated here; at a physical level, it is linked to the Islets of Langerhans in the pancreas; its energies also affect the solar and splenic nerve plexuses, the digestive system, the pancreas, liver, gall bladder, diaphragm and middle back
Imbalance	people who are under stress will show imbalance in this chakra; shock and stress have a greater impact on this chakra; it is in the solar plexus chakra that negative energies relating to thoughts and feelings are processed; people with an imbalance in this chakra may feel depressed, insecure, lacking in confidence and may worry what others think
Colour association	yellow

The Heart Chakra

Location	in the centre of the chest
Relevance	concerned with love and the heart; it deals with all issues concerned with love and affection; at a physical level it is linked to the thymus gland; its energies also affect the cardiac and pulmonary nerve plexuses, the heart, lungs, bronchial tubes, chest, upper back and arms; the point of connection between the upper and lower chakras
Imbalance	if the energy does not flow freely between the solar plexus and the heart, or between the heart and the throat, it can lead to energy withdrawal into the body; a person with an imbalance in this chakra may feel sorry for themselves, be afraid of letting go, feel unworthy of love or feel terrified of rejection
Colour association	green

The Throat Chakra

Location	at the base of the neck
Relevance	concerned with communication and expression, it also deals with the issue of truth and true expression of the soul; at a physical level, it is linked to the thyroid and parathyroid glands; its energies also affect the pharyngeal nerve plexus, the organs of the throat, the neck, nose, mouth, teeth and ears
Imbalance	if this chakra is out of balance it may affect our ability to express our emotions, frustration and tension may result; a person with an imbalance in this chakra may feel unable to relax
Colour association	blue

The Brow Chakra

Location	in the middle of the forehead over the third eye area
Relevance	commonly known as the 'third eye', the brow chakra is the storehouse of memories and imagination and is associated with intellect, understanding and intuition; at a physical level, it is linked to the hypothalamus and pituitary gland; its energies also affect the nerves of the head, brain, eyes and face
Imbalance	if this chakra is not functioning correctly it can lead to headaches and nightmares; a person with an imbalance in this chakra may be oversensitive, be afraid of success, be non-assertive and undisciplined
Colour association	indigo

The Crown Chakra

Location	on top of the head
Relevance	the centre of our spirituality and is concerned with thinking and decision-making; at a physical level it is linked to the pineal gland; its energies also affect the brain and the rest of the body
Imbalance	an imbalance in this chakra may be reflected in an unwillingness to open up to our spiritual potential; an imbalance may also show in an inability to make decisions
Colour association	violet

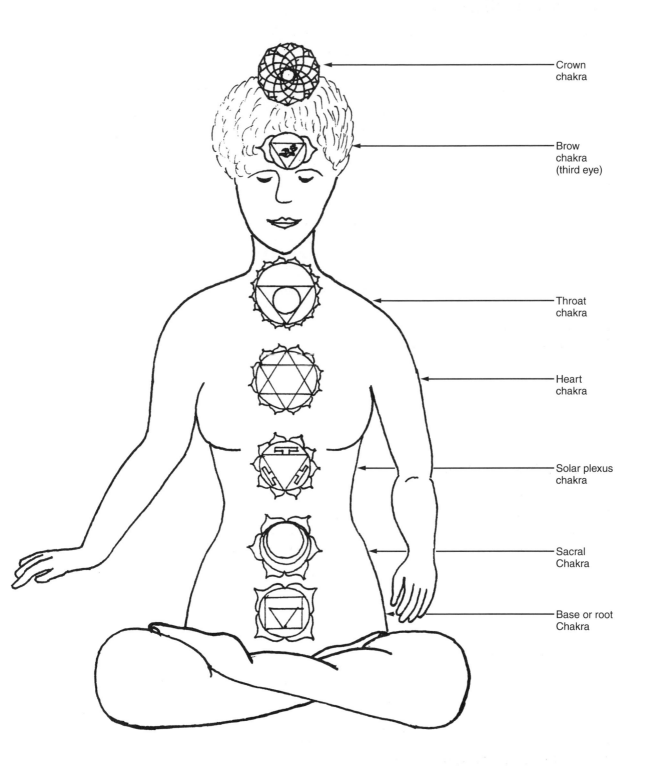

Crown chakra

Brow chakra (third eye)

Throat chakra

Heart chakra

Solar plexus chakra

Sacral Chakra

Base or root Chakra

Figure 4.12 The chakras

CHAPTER 5
Therapeutic massage therapy

INTRODUCTION

Massage can be defined as the systematic and manual manipulation of the soft tissues of the body in order to promote health and well-being. It is an ancient art that has been practised and performed for many thousands of years – well before the advent of medicine or surgery. Today, it is a multi-dimensional skill encompassing a wide variety of ever evolving techniques.

Massage has evolved from a combination of eastern and western traditions. However, in recent years the basic forms of massage have been extended and added to with a number of other specialised techniques. Massage is a natural way of maintaining the vital human connection: touch. It also extends beyond fulfilling the need for touch, as it has many health benefits; a major application is in relieving stress. In addition, it is a powerful healing tool that enhances physical and emotional health, as it improves the circulation of nutrients to the body and encourages the body to heal itself.

BRIEF HISTORY

Massage is ancient in origin and is embedded in human culture. The earliest evidence for the use of massage is found in cave drawings and paintings which demonstrate the use of touch as a form of healing. Prehistoric artefacts suggest that ancient cultures practised the rubbing of herbs on the body.

China

The Chinese were the first to practice massage to help treat illness and maintain health. As long ago as 3000BC they used a combination of herbs, exercise and massage on particular parts of the body, known as 'amma'. This is described in a book called the *Cong Fau of Tao Tsu*. Massage still features as an important part of health maintenance in China. The modern term for massage in China is 'Tui-na'.

India

Massage has been practised in India for over 3000 years. A sacred Hindu text called the *Ayur-Veda* (*The Art of Life*), written around 1800 BC lists massage as one of its *principles of hygiene*. Other Hindu texts contain descriptions of 'tshanpau', or massage at the bath, and describes how shampooing and rubbing was used to promote well-being, as well as for hygiene. Techniques also included kneading, tapping, friction, anointing the body with perfumes, and cracking the joints of the neck, fingers and toes.

Egypt

The Egyptians used massage for its therapeutic and cosmetic effects, and Egyptian tombs show evidence of pots and jars used to mix oils, fats, herbs and resins.

Japan

Around the sixth century AD the techniques introduced by the Chinese were adopted by the Japanese, who named the parts on the body outlined by 'amma' as 'tsubo' points. These techniques were further developed to form a method of finger pressure called shiatsu which includes manipulation of chi. Shiatsu is now being practised by many therapists.

Greece

The ancient Greeks advocated the benefits of massage on health. Aesculapius, a Greek physician and priest developed a system of gymnastics which was made up of a combination of exercise and massage. Massage was used before sporting events to help improve performance and to aid recovery from injury and fatigue. The gymnasium founded by Aesculapius (the first of its kind) became a place to learn, exercise, discuss philosophy, have massage for health, beauty and healing. Around 500 BC the Greek physician Herodicus used oils with herbs for massage in order to help treat medical conditions.

Hippocrates, known as the 'father of holistic medicine' and a pupil of Herodicus, began studying the effects of massage on the body. Hippocrates discovered that massage was more beneficial when applied in a direction towards the heart, although the circulatory system was not fully understood then. He taught massage techniques to his pupils and advised that 'a physician must be experienced in many things but assuredly in rubbing'. He also wrote that 'rubbing can bind a joint that is too rigid ... Hard rubbing binds, much rubbing causes parts to waste and moderate rubbing makes them grow'.

The Romans

The Romans adopted many aspects of Greek culture. In doing so, they acquired the art of massage as a medical treatment for many conditions, as well as for hygiene.

The Roman Emperor, Marcus Aurelius's renowned physician Galen prescribed massage for injured gladiators. He wrote many books relating to the value of massage and exercise. He talked of 'pommelling, squeezing and pinching' the muscles and experimented with the direction of massage movements, according to individual needs. Large public baths were built to include wet areas with water baths and steam rooms and dry areas for massage and a gymnasium.

Very little is recorded of massage between the decline of the Roman Empire (around 500 AD) and the early Middle Ages (around 1400AD). At this time, appropriately called the Dark Ages, massage was considered evil and sinful. Despite this, the practice of massage did persist throughout the Middle Ages, largely due to an Islamic philosopher, physician and writer known as Rhazes, who was a dedicated follower of Hippocrates. He wrote an encyclopaedia of Arabic, Roman and Greek medical practices advocating the value of massage as a means to treat and prevent disease.

Massage in Modern Times

Sixteenth-century physicians began using massage in the treatment of their patients. A French physician, Ambroise Pare, reputedly helped restore Mary Queen of Scots's health through massage. From then on, massage became established as a form of medical therapy.

By far the greatest advancement of therapeutic massage recorded in history was by a Swedish physiologist called Per Henrik Ling (1776–1839). Ling established an Institute for researching massage and called the system of techniques he developed 'medical gymnastics'. This was based on active and passive exercises and a series of massage movements. He introduced French terms such as 'effleurage', 'petrissage', 'friction', 'vibration' and through his research, and a considerable amount of practical experience, he created a scientific system of therapeutic massage known as Swedish Massage.

Dr Johann Mezgner of Holland adapted massage techniques based on his knowledge of anatomy and physiology. His theory of massage, which was based on scientific principles, became accepted as part of medical practice in Germany, Denmark, Norway and North America.

In 1894, a group of women established The Society of Trained Masseuses, as the demand for trained massage therapists grew. In 1920, it was amalgamated with the Institute of Massage and Remedial exercise and was later registered in 1943 as the Chartered Society of Physiotherapy. In 1964 physiotherapy became established as a state registered profession.

As electrical equipment started to supersede manual massage in physiotherapy, the use of massage to treat medical conditions started to decline. However, this still left a need for massage in clinics, health farms and leisure centres, as people were becoming more aware of the benefits of massage to their general well-being.

Today massage has developed into a combination of techniques which all have their roots in the Swedish system. As the public image of massage has changed over the past 10 years, there are now more opportunities for massage therapists to work alongside other health care professionals, in hospitals and hospices and for sports teams and clubs. Massage has stood the test of time due to its inherent value. At the beginning of the twenty-first century more and more people are realising the importance of massage as an antidote to stress and as an aid to good health.

BENEFITS AND EFFECTS

In order to understand the benefits of massage, it is important to consider how the body responds physiologically.

Massage involves two types of responses:
- mechanical responses as a result of pressure and movement as the soft tissues are manipulated
- reflex responses in which the nerves respond to stimulation.

The Physiological Effects of Massage

Effects on the Skeletal System
- Massage can help increase joint mobility by reducing any thickening of the connective tissue and helping to release restrictions in the fascia.
- It helps to free adhesions, break down scar tissue and decrease inflammation. As a result it can restore a range of motion to stiff joints.
- Massage improves muscle tone and balance, reducing the physical stress placed on bones and joints.

Effects on the Muscular System
- Massage relieves muscular tightness, stiffness, spasms and restrictions in the muscle tissue.
- It increase flexibility in muscles due to muscular relaxation.
- It increases blood circulation bringing more oxygen and nutrients into the muscle. This reduces muscle fatigue and soreness.
- It promotes rapid removal of toxins and waste products from the muscle.

Effects on the Cardiovascular System
Massage can:
- improve circulation by mechanically assisting the venous flow of blood back to the heart
- dilate blood vessels helping them to work more efficiently
- produce an enhanced blood flow–delivery of fresh oxygen and nutrients to the tissues is improved and the removal of waste products, toxins and carbon dioxide is hastened via the venous system
- help temporarily to decrease blood pressure, due to dilation of capillaries
- create hyperaemia (erythema) resulting from the increased blood flow
- decrease the heart rate due to relaxation and the decreased stimulation of the sympathetic nervous system
- reduce ischemia (ischemia is a reduction in the flow of blood to body parts, often marked by pain and tissue dysfunction).

Effects on the Lymphatic System

Massage helps to:

■ reduce oedema by increasing lymphatic drainage and the removal of waste from the system

■ regular massage may help to strengthen the immune system, due to the increase in white blood cells.

Effects on the Nervous System

■ Massage stimulates sensory receptors; this can either stimulate or soothe nerves depending on the techniques used.

■ It also stimulates the parasympathetic nervous system, helping promote relaxation and the reduction of stress.

■ Massage helps to reduce pain by the release of endorphins (endorphins are also known to elevate the mood).

Effects on the Skin

Massage can bring about:

■ improved circulation to the skin, increasing nutrition to the cells and encouraging cell regeneration

■ increased production of sweat from the sweat glands, helping to excrete urea and waste products through the skin

■ vaso-dilation of the surface capillaries helping to improve the skin's colour

■ desquamation

■ improved elasticity of the skin

■ increased sebum production, helping to improve the skin's suppleness and resistance to infection.

Effects on the Respiratory System

■ Massage deepens respiration and improves lung capacity by relaxing any tightness in the respiratory muscles.

■ It also slows down the rate of respiration due to the reduced stimulation of the sympathetic nervous system.

Effects on the Digestive System

Massage can:

■ increase peristalsis in the large intestine, helping to relieve constipation, colic and gas

■ promote the activity of the parasympathetic nervous system, which stimulates digestion.

Effects on the Urinary System

■ Massage increases urinary output due to the increased circulation and lymph drainage from the tissues.

The Psychological Effects of Massage

Massage can help to:

- reduce stress and anxiety by relaxing both mind and body
- create a feeling of well-being and enhanced self-esteem
- promote positive body awareness and an improved body image through relaxation
- ease emotional trauma through relaxation and relief of repressed feelings.

PREPARATION FOR MASSAGE

About the Equipment

A successful massage treatment is not only dependent on the skill and knowledge of the therapist, but on the therapist's ability to use the tools of the trade correctly. Correct choice of equipment for massage is important to ensure comfort for both the therapist and the client.

The Treatment Couch

Treatment couches for massage may be static or portable. Portable couches are becoming more popular due to their versatility and because they save space.

- **Height** – the optimum height for the massage couch is determined by the height of the therapist and the therapy being practised. In order to determine the correct height, the therapist should stand at the side of the couch and be able to place the flat of the hand on the couch with the arm extended. Portable massage couches with an adjustable height range are useful for different types of therapies and different sized clients.
- **Width** – massage couches come in a range of standard widths although manufacturers will custom build couches to special requirements. In most cases, the width of the couch will depend on the height of the therapist and the frame size of the client. If the couch is too wide it may difficult to reach across. Larger clients may find it uncomfortable to lie on a narrow couch if their arms hang off the sides. Side extensions can be added to some couches to increase the width of the top end.
- **Length** – most couches are six feet long. This may be increased by the use of a table extension fitted to the head or foot end of the couch – useful for a tall client.
- **Frame** – couch frames are either made of wood or aluminium. The major difference is that aluminium frames are stronger.
- **Padding** – the padding determines the comfort level for the client. Some couches are made with a single layer of foam and some are multi-layered, offering a deeper, more luxurious feel. It is very important to ensure that the padding is fire retardant for health and safety reasons.
- **Fabric** – the foam padding is usually covered with vinyl, as it is long lasting and easy to clean. The vinyl should be cleaned and disinfected regularly with a mild cleaning detergent. Avoid products with alcohol or bleach as these may erode the vinyl. Care should be taken to ensure that the vinyl fabric does not get too hot or too cold. This is particularly important if you are a visiting therapist and you leave the couch in your car.

Couch Accessories

There are many optional extras which can increase the versatility of the massage couch, increase client comfort and improve the ease of movement for the therapist.

- **Multi-position backrest** – this can improve the versatility of the massage couch. Occasionally, clients may be unable to lay flat or may wish to sit up after their massage. The backrest is adjustable and allows the therapist to select the most comfortable position for the client.
- **Face holes** – this is a hole which may be incorporated into the main body of the couch. Sometimes, the face hole is provided with a flap which can be closed. Face holes enable the client to keep their neck straight if they find this more comfortable. However, some clients find face holes claustrophobic.
- **Face cradles** – similar to a face hole but less claustrophobic, a face rest or cradle allows the client to keep their head an neck straight whilst lying prone and can increase their comfort. It can also facilitate access to the client's head, neck and shoulders. Some manufacturers offer adjustable face cradles – the angle may be adjusted to suit the client and the type of holistic therapy being practised.
- **Bolsters** – bolsters are designed to enhance client comfort and to give support. Bolsters may be placed under the ankles of a prone client, or under the knees when lying supine. A face cushion is practical when using a face hole to support the client's head and neck.

About Massage Lubricants

Massage media include oils, creams and talc. A good massage medium will nourish the skin and allow a free-flowing movement.

> **KEY NOTE** When choosing a massage medium, it is important to consider how a client's skin may react. Some clients may be sensitive to certain products. If a client has as history of allergies and sensitivity, care should be taken to discuss potential allergens and to avoid products which could sensitise the client's skin.

The amount of lubricant used will be determined partly by the client's skin type and partly by the client's preference. Massage mediums may be scented or unscented. Care should be taken to consider any allergies before using a scented product. As some clients may find the smell of perfumed products offensive, you should allow them to smell a scented medium before proceeding.

During the initial consultation, it is important to establish whether the client has sensitive skin or a history of allergies. If this is the case, you should carry out a **patch test**. A patch test involves washing the area of the inner bend of the elbow with a mild soap and warm water. Rinse the area and then apply a small amount of the product intended for use on the skin. Allow between 15 and 30 minutes to see if there is a reaction, such as signs of itching, inflammation and sensitivity or stinging. If so, do not use the product.

Types of Massage Media

■ **Oil** – this is the most common form of lubricant used in massage as it allows the hands to glide over the area. It is preferable to use massage oils that nourish the skin such as grapeseed, almond, apricot kernel, peach kernel, safflower, sunflower and coconut.

> **KEY NOTE** There are many prepared massage blends which may be scented with aromatic oils or perfumes. Care should be taken to establish the ingredients before using, to avoid adverse reactions.
>
> The use of minerals oils is not recommended for massage as they are petroleum-based and tend to dry the skin, deplete nutrients and clog the pores. You should avoid nut-based oils if the client suffers from a nut allergy.

■ **Cream** – massage creams are more emollient (smoothing and softening) and less greasy than massage oil. They have the added benefits of nourishing and softening the skin, and being more readily absorbed. The disadvantage of using cream as a massage medium is that it absorbs into the skin more quickly than oil. The therapist may need to apply cream frequently throughout the massage to avoid dragging the skin. Massage cream is suitable for all skin types but may be preferred for dry skins.

■ **Talc** – talcum powder is a dry lubricant for clients who dislike the feeling of oil on their skin or any lubricant that leave a residue. Talc is also suitable for clients with oily skin or for those who perspire easily. Care should be taken when applying talcum powder to the skin as small particles may enter the nasal passages and cause the client or therapist to cough or sneeze

Preparation of the Massage Couch

Before preparing the massage couch, the therapist should check the height, and that the equipment is safe for use. Look for rivets or fixings that may have become loose.

The couch may be covered with a protective towelling sheet and covered in couch roll from head to foot. Some therapists prefer to cover the towelling sheet with towels, instead of using couch roll. However, this will increase the cost of laundry, as towels must be replaced for each client. There should be a plentiful supply of towels for covering the client; a bath sheet and a couple of additional smaller towels.

Pillows or head supports may be used and should be covered with a protective covering and a towel. Small towels, wrapped in disposable tissue, may be used to make bolsters or limb supports for placing under the ankles when the client is prone, and under the knees when supine.

A stool should be placed under the couch and a piece of tissue placed on the floor. This is for the client to step onto after they have removed their shoes. A small, lined bin should be placed under the couch. This is used for all waste materials and to avoid the risk of contamination.

Trolley Preparation

The trolley should be prepared with all the necessary materials *before* the client arrives. It should be positioned for ease of access and used. The trolley should be cleaned and lined with disposable couch roll.

The following items should be displayed on the top of the trolley:
- a bottle of surgical spirit for cleansing the client's feet
- a variety of massage mediums – massage oil, talc and cream – it is preferable to use pump dispensers to avoid the risk of contamination
- disposable spatulas
- a bowl containing cotton wool
- tissues
- a spare bowl for the client's jewellery or accessories (for safety and security the client may prefer to place their valuables in their handbag, or with their personal belongings)
- a bottle of cologne to remove excess oil from the client's skin
- spare sheets of couch roll
- massage props and bolsters
- spare towels which may be placed on the lower shelf of the trolley.

Preparing the Environment

A comfortable and relaxing atmosphere for massage can be created by considering the following factors:
- **Lighting** – this should be soft and discreet; avoid bright, overhead lighting.
- **Temperature** – the massage environment should be comfortably warm (between 68–75 °F, 20–24 °C). If the treatment room is too cold or too hot, it may inhibit client relaxation. Due to activation of the parasympathetic nervous system, the body cools down during massage.
- **Ventilation** – the atmosphere should be well ventilated and free from draughts in order to keep the environment fresh and healthy.
- **Decor and colours** – it is preferable to choose colours that add warmth and give the impression of comfort, rather than harsh colours which are too dark or too bright.
- **Privacy** – a massage treatment room should always be private to ensure client relaxation. A movable curtain or screen may be used to create a cubicle.
- **Atmosphere and noise level** – relaxation tapes can create a calming atmosphere for massage. A therapist should always ask the client if they would like music (some people prefer quite) and, ideally, there should be a choice of tapes to suit different tastes.

Preparation of the Therapist

Remember that first impressions are very important. The first impression may determine whether the client comes back for treatments on a regular basis. In order to project a professional image in the workplace, therapists should pay attention to the following factors:

- **Professional workwear** – clothes should be clean, freshly laundered and ironed, and should project an image of professionalism.
- **Footwear** – shoes should be low-heeled or flat, and comfortable; massage can be very tiring and is physically demanding.
- **Hair** – hair should be tied back neatly if long, and presented in a well groomed style.
- **Jewellery** – no obtrusive jewellery should be worn as it may scratch or irritate a client's skin; rings with stones or sharp edges should be avoided, as these may injure the client and can harbour bacteria. Therapists should remove face and nose rings in order to project a professional image.
- **Hands and nails** – hands should be kept as soft as possible and must be protected from harsh chemicals. Nails should be kept short, clean and without nail enamel. Hands should also be cleansed and warm before commencing a massage.
- **Avoid wearing strong perfumes or scented lotions** – it is important to avoid strong smells which may be offensive to the client; respect a client's susceptibility to allergies and sensitisation.
- **Personal hygiene** – due to the close nature of the work, personal hygiene is of paramount importance. Therapists should bath or shower daily and use and effective antiperspirant or deodorant, as necessary. Avoid consuming food that may cause an offensive odour and brush teeth regularly.

Learn Correct Body Mechanics

Body mechanics involves the correct use of posture in order to apply massage with the maximum efficiency and the minimal trauma to the therapist.

> **KEY NOTE** As well as increasing the effectiveness of the massage, the use of correct body mechanics helps to prevent repetitive strain injuries, decrease fatigue and increases comfort for the therapist.

Guidelines for correct body mechanics include:

- Check the couch height – a couch at the correct height will enable the therapist to use their body weight effectively to develop pressure. Other considerations are the size of the client (larger clients will generally require a lower couch height) and the type of therapy being performed.
- Warm up before a massage.
- Wear low-healed shoes with good support.
- Keep the back straight by tilting the pelvis forwards.
- Use the body weight effectively, by lunging in order to create pressure.
- Keep the shoulders and upper back relaxed (avoiding raising shoulders towards the ears).
- Keep feet placed firmly on the ground.
- Bend the knees slightly and keep them soft, taking care to avoid locking them straight.
- Keep wrists as straight as possible.
- Avoid joint hyperextension.

■ Keep arms perpendicular to the upper body and forearms parallel to the ground, whenever possible.

■ Avoid reaching over the massage table (this may strain the back).

■ Keep the body in correct alignment by maintaining the head erect over the neck and shoulders.

■ Keep the head forward posture to a minimum and avoid spending too much time looking down.

■ Take breaks in between clients to stretch the neck, shake out the arms and relax.

■ Vary the massage techniques used and alter the hand and foot placements.

■ Have regular massage treatments in order to keep body working at an optimum level.

CAUTIONS AND CONTRA-INDICATIONS FOR MASSAGE THERAPY

It is important, in order to safeguard the health of the client and to protect the therapist, that contra-indications are discussed with the client during the consultation. Any restrictions to the massage treatment should be clearly and tactfully explained to the client.

In certain cases, it may be necessary to refer the client to their GP before treatment is applied. Where possible, treatment should be adapted to suit the client's condition and needs.

■ **Fever** – this is a contra-indication due to the risk of spreading infection as a result of increased circulation. During fever, the body temperature rises as a result of infection.

■ **Infectious disease** (e.g. colds, flu, measles, mumps, tuberculosis, scarlet fever) – these are contra-indicated due to the fact they are highly contagious.

■ **Skin diseases** – care should be taken as contagious conditions may be spread by the massage. If the condition is infectious then massage should be avoided due to the risk of cross infection.

■ **Recent haemorrhage** – haemorrhage is excessive bleeding which may be either internal or external. Massage should be avoided due to increasing the risk of blood spillage from blood vessels.

■ **Severe circulatory disorders and heart conditions** – medical clearance should always be sought before massaging a client with a severe heart condition or circulatory problem, as the increased circulation from the massage may overburden the heart and can increase the risk of a thrombus or embolus.

KEY NOTE If medical clearance is given, massage should be applied lightly and gently.

■ **Thrombosis** – always seek medical clearance before massaging a client with a history of thrombosis or embolism as there is a risk that the increased circulation may move the clot to the heart, lungs or brain.

> **KEY NOTE** If medical clearance is given, massage should be applied lightly and gently.

■ **High blood pressure** – clients with high blood pressure should have medical referral prior to massage, even if they are on prescribed medication, due to their susceptibility to thrombosis. Clients on anti-hypertensive medication may be prone to postural hypotension and may feel light headed and dizzy after treatment. Care should, therefore, be taken to assist a client off the couch and ensure that they get up slowly.

> **KEY NOTE** Once clearance is granted, massage should be soothing and relaxing.

■ **Low blood pressure** – clients suffering from low blood pressure may experience dizziness when sitting or standing up after massage and could fall.
■ **Epilepsy** – due to the complexity of the condition, medical advice should always be sought before massaging a client who has a history of epilepsy. There is a theoretical risk that over-stimulation or deep relaxation may provoke a convulsion (although this has never been proven in practice).

> **KEY NOTE** As some types of epilepsy may be triggered by smells, care should be taken with the choice of medium used.

■ **Diabetes** – this is a condition which requires medical referral, as clients with diabetes may be prone to arteriosclerosis, high blood pressure and oedema. Pressure should be monitored and administered carefully. If the client has any loss in sensory nerve function they will be unable to give accurate feedback regarding pressure.

> **KEY NOTE** If the client is receiving insulin by injection, care should be taken to avoid massage on recent injection sites. Clients should have their medication with them when they attend for treatment, in case of an emergency.

- **Cancer** – medical clearance should always be sought before massaging a client with a cancerous condition. There is a risk of certain types of cancer spreading through the lymphatic system; massage is also thought to aid in the metasis of the cancer. It is unlikely that gentle massage can cause cancer to spread through the stimulation of lymph flow, however it is important to obtain advice from the consultant or medical team concerning the type of cancer and the extent of the disease. Once medical clearance has been given, massage may help to relax the body and support the immune system. It may also be used in **palliative care** (therapy that eases or reduces pain and other symptoms).
- **Skin disorders** – care should be taken as the condition may be worsened. Some skins conditions such as eczema, dermatitis and psoriasis should be treated as a localised contra-indication. Areas may be hypersensitive and the condition may be exacerbated by massage.
- **Recent scar tissue** – massage should only be applied once the tissue is fully healed and can withstand pressure. Massage, in particular gentle friction movements, may be applied over healed scar tissue in order to help break down adhesions.
- **Severe bruising** – localised massage is contra-indicated in order to avoid discomfort and pain.
- **Varicose veins** – these should be treated as a localised contra-indication. Clients with varicose veins may be prone to thromboses and, therefore, clearance from their GP may be necessary. Massage should not be applied directly over the affected area, but gentle massage may be given close to the area in order to reduce oedema and prevent venous and lymphatic stasis.

KEY NOTE When massaging a cancer patient, always avoid massage over areas of the body receiving radiation therapy, close to tumour sites and areas of skin cancer. It is usual to offer short, light massage to certain parts of the body such as the hands, face and feet.

- **Cuts and abrasions** – these should be avoided as massage could further damage the healing tissue and expose the client and therapist to infection.

KEY NOTE When massaging a client with varicose veins, ideally their legs should be raised above their heart during treatment.

- **Recent fractures** – these should be treated as a localised contra-indication in order not to interfere with the healing process. There is a danger of inflammation and causing damage. Always seek medical clearance before massaging.

- **Recent sprains or injuries** – it is important to wait for at least 72 hours before massaging a minor injury or sprain, due to the risk of increased vascular bleeding. Ice may be applied to the injured area once medical clearance is received.
- **Undiagnosed lumps, bumps and swellings** – the client should be referred to their GP for a diagnosis. Massage may increase the susceptibility to damage in the area by virtue of the pressure and motion.

Special Factors to Take into Consideration Before Massaging

- **Asthma** – care should be taken to position the client comfortably (usually semi-reclining) and to avoid using any massage mediums or substances that the client may be allergic to.
- **Allergies** – care should be taken to ensure that massage products and the treatment room do not contain anything to which the client may be allergic. Patch tests should be carried out to avoid hypersensitisation and adverse reactions to products.
- **Medications** – it is important to take care when massaging someone who is on prescribed or over-the-counter drugs that reduce pain, distort their responses or impair their ability to give feedback. It is advisable to refer the client to their GP to establish why the medication is being taken and to ensure their suitability for treatment.
- **Pregnancy** – avoid any form of massage in the early stages of pregnancy and, thereafter, avoid deep massage over the abdominal area.
- **Abdominal treatment for women during menstruation** – the abdominal area should be omitted from the massage treatment during menstruation to avoid discomfort; some clients find that massaging the lower back provides comfort and helps to relieve pain.

CLIENT CONSULTATION RECORDS FOR THERAPEUTIC MASSAGE THERAPY

A consultation for massage therapy will cover the following areas:
- the client's medical history and any current medical treatment
- general state of health
- lifestyle patterns
- any presenting problems
- client declaration and signature.

Therapists should be tactful when explaining any restrictions to the massage treatment or the reasons for a referral to the GP.

An example of a massage therapy consultation form is given overleaf. See page 10 for a client referral form if required.

BODY MASSAGE CONSULTATION FORM

Client Note

The following information is required for your safety and to benefit your health. Whilst massage is totally safe when administered professionally by a trained massage therapist, there are certain conditions which may require special care. The following details will be treated in the strictest of confidence. It may, however, be necessary for you to consult your GP before any massage treatment can be given.

Date of initial consultation:_____   Client ref. No. _____

Personal Details

Name: _____   Title: Mr/Mrs/Miss/Ms/Other

Address: _____

_____

Telephone Number _____   Daytime: _____   Evening: _____

Date of Birth: _____   Occupation:_____

Medical details

Name of Doctor: _____   Surgery: _____

Address: _____

_____

Telephone Number: _____

Do you have/have you ever suffered with any of the following conditions?
(Please give dates and details)

			Dates and Details
High or low blood pressure	Y	N	_____
Heart condition	Y	N	_____
Thrombosis	Y	N	_____
Varicose veins or phlebitis	Y	N	_____
Dysfunction of the nervous system	Y	N	_____
Recent injury	Y	N	_____
Any type of infectious conditions	Y	N	_____
Recent fractures or sprains	Y	N	_____
Arthritis	Y	N	_____
Diabetes	Y	N	_____
Epilepsy	Y	N	_____
Asthma	Y	N	_____
Skin diseases or disorders	Y	N	_____

Recent haemorrhage	Y	N	_____
Abdominal or digestive complaint or hernia	Y	N	_____
Do you have any serious conditions such as cancer or tumours?	Y	N	_____
Do you have any recent scar tissue/bruises/ open cuts/large moles/lumps/other swellings?	Y	N	_____
Do you suffer from any allergies?	Y	N	_____

Female Clients

Is it possible that you may be pregnant?	Y	N	_____
If pregnant, how many months (any complications)?	Y	N	_____
Are you currently menstruating?	Y	N	_____

Current medical treatment: _____

_____

_____

Current medication (list dosages): _____

_____

Section for use by therapist
GP referral required: Yes ( )   No ( )
Clearance form sent: Yes ( )   No ( )   Date:_____
Clearance form received: Yes ( )   No ( )   Date:_____

General State of Health and Lifestyle

Do you smoke?   Yes ( ) average per day _____   No ( )

Do you drink alcohol?   Yes ( ) average daily consumption _____   No ( )

How many glasses of water do you drink daily? _____

How would you describe your diet? _____

Stress levels: High ( )   Medium ( )   Low ( )

Sleep pattern: Good ( )   Average ( )   Poor ( )

Exercise undertaken/lifestyle: _____

_____

Do you follow a regular exercise programme?   Yes ( )   No ( )

_____

Details_____

_____

Do you have any hobbies/time set aside for relaxation?   Yes ( )   No ( )

Details_____

_____

Have you ever had a massage treatment before?   Yes ( )   No ( )

If yes, please give brief details of previous treatments and success: _____

_____

Are you currently having any other forms of alternative or complementary therapy treatment? (please state) _____

_____

Client Declaration

I declare that the information that I have given, is true and correct and that, as far as I am aware, I can undertake treatment with this establishment without any adverse effects. I have been fully informed about contra-indications and am willing, therefore, to proceed. I understand that massage therapy is not a substitute for medical advice and/or treatment.

Client's signature: _____   Date: _____

Therapist's signature: _____   Date: _____

TREATMENT-PLANNING AND RECORD-KEEPING FOR MASSAGE TREATMENTS

Treatment planning is an essential part of practice as its takes account of the client's individual needs for each treatment session. A treatment plan for massage therapy will typically include the following information:
- the date of treatment
- feedback from any previous treatments (if applicable), noting the client's response and any changes or improvements in the client's condition
- any new information relating to the client's condition and which is required to update the original consultation form
- the treatment objectives for the session and any specific client needs
- an outline plan of the proposed treatment to include areas for treatment, the length of the treatment and the cost.

In addition to the above information, it is important for the massage therapist to record the following on the client's treatment record:
- the type of medium used

- a manual and visual evaluation of the client's tissues, noting any areas of tension, erythema, areas of fluid retention, adhesions and fibrosis etc.
- any known contra-actions, their effects on the client and the advice given
- after care advice given
- home care advice given, along with any products recommended
- outcome and evaluation of the treatment
- recommendations for future treatment.

PREPARATION OF THE CLIENT

- **Guidance and explanation** – it is important to explain carefully the massage procedure to the client. New clients may feel nervous and apprehensive when attending for a massage. It is important to allow time for clients to ask questions about the treatment. The therapist should reassure the client so that they can then relax and enjoy their massage.
- **Clothing removal** – when clients attend for massage for this first time, they should be told how much clothing to remove (it is considered hygienic for the client to retain their underpants). It is important to respect a client's modesty and privacy when undressing and to provide a suitably private area for changing. Once a client has undressed, they may be advised to wrap a large, bath sheet-sized towel around them.
- **Removal of jewellery and accessories** – clients should be advised to remove all obtrusive jewellery and accessories which may inhibit the flow of the massage. Clients should remove spectacles and clients who wear contact lenses may wish to remove them in case they start to feel uncomfortable. It is important for the therapist to hand spectacles back to the client before they get off the couch, to avoid risk of falls.
- **Hair** – if the client's hair is long, use a hair covering or ask the client to tie their hair up.
- **Covering the client** – the primary concerns here are for client modesty and client comfort. When massaging, it is important to ensure that only the body areas being massaged are exposed. Covering body parts keeps the client warm and creates a physical and psychological boundary, giving the client a feeling of security and privacy.
- **Assisting the client on and off the couch** – for reasons of safety, the therapist should assist the client on and off the massage couch. If the couch is too high or the client has a disability, a foot stool may be useful.

Client Positioning

It is important for the therapist to position correctly and support the client for massage treatment. This ensures the client is comfortable and relaxed to receive the treatment and helps the therapist to work effectively and prevent injuries to themselves.

Once the client has been helped onto the couch, they should be covered by one large bath sheet laid lengthways and another bath towel laid sideways. When lying prone, the client may be offered a face hole or face cradle and a face cushion keep their neck straight. Props may be positioned under the ankles in order to help support the back. The client's arms may be placed alongside their body or on either side of the head. When lying supine, props may be placed under the knees and a cushion may be provided to support the head and neck.

REQUIREMENTS FOR AN EFFECTIVE MASSAGE

■ **Well trained hands** – hands should be supple and flexible to practice massage effectively. In order to increase sensitivity and flexibility, it is advisable to exercise the hands and wrists regularly.

■ **Correct stance and posture** – good posture and proper body alignment is essential whilst performing a massage treatment as this allows the therapist to utilise their body weight effectively for maximum depth of pressure. Correct posture allows the therapist to develop an even rhythm and freedom of movement, and prevents back, joint and muscular strain. There are two main stances for massage:

1. **Walk standing** – this is the position a therapist assumes when working longitudinally down the length of the muscle, with one foot in front of the other (the therapist's head faces the client's head). When assuming this position, the therapist lunges forward into the strokes with the front knee slightly bent, rather than leaning over and bending the back.

2. **Stride standing** – this is the position a therapist assumes when working transversely across the muscles. The therapist should be facing the couch with their feet slightly apart. For general points on posture and body alignment see pages 81–82 on body mechanics.

■ **Pressure** – the pressure of movements applied will vary according to the type of tissue being massaged, the areas being treated and the client's preference. The application of

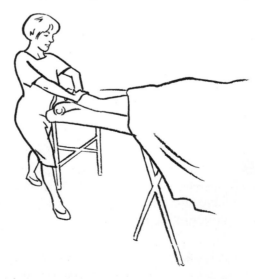

Figure 5.1 Walk standing posture

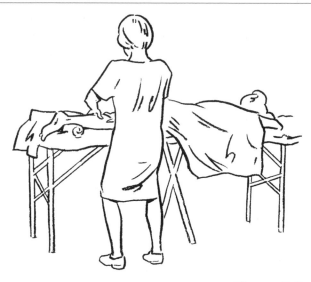

Figure 5.2 Stride standing posture

correct pressure is aided largely by the transference of body weight through the arms and shoulders into the hands, and through lunging into the strokes.

■ **Even rhythm** – In order to establish a rhythmic massage, the movements should be applied continuously and consistently. It is important to avoid breaking contact during a massage as this affects the continuity and rhythm. It is difficult for clients to relax if the massage lacks a smooth rhythm and continuity. Care should be taken, therefore, to ensure that the therapist's hands are relaxed and flexible, the therapist's positioning is correct and the height of the couch is correct.

■ **Correct rate** – the rate of massage movements will be determined by the purpose of the massage. In general, a faster rate of massage will stimulate and a slower rate will sedate and relax. If a massage is too fast, it may cause tension and fatigue, and the client will not be able to relax. In addition to this, the therapist may be unable to assess the soft tissues. Therapeutic massage is generally performed at a moderately slow speed.

■ **Breathing** – correct breathing is important for both the therapist and the client during a massage. In order to give a good massage, a therapist should be relaxed; breathing deeply and slowly will help to aid relaxation.

■ **Attitude** – massage involves the transference of energy and in order to give a good

KEY NOTE Breathing deeply throughout a massage can help the lungs to function more efficiently. It ensures that all the body's cells receive an adequate amount of oxygen and dispose of enough carbon dioxide. When the body is under stress, the chest muscles become tense and breathing tends to be very shallow. If the abdominal muscles are tense, the diaphragm is unable to expand fully or relax and, over a period of time, breathing will suffer. Deep breathing should, therefore, be encouraged throughout a massage to help regulate breathing patterns and to aid deep relaxation.

massage, the therapist should be relaxed and in right frame of mind. The wrong attitude to this type of work can be easily detected by the client.

PRE-MASSAGE OR PRE-HEAT TREATMENTS

Thermotherapy or pre-heat treatments involve the external application of heat for therapeutic purposes. There are several types of pre-heating treatment that may be used prior to massage including:

- paraffin wax
- infra-red light
- audio-sonic
- heat-inducing products.

There are benefits to using heat treatments prior to massage:

- Heat treatments stimulate and increase blood volume, providing the tissues with increased oxygen and nutrition.
- Blood vessels near the skin's surface begin to dilate and create a flushed appearance due to hyperaemia.
- They help to relax muscular tension and spams by softening the fascia.
- They soothe and relax the client.
- Heat helps to alleviate pain.
- By raising the temperature, heat treatments stimulate perspiration through the sweat glands.

Paraffin Wax

This technique is used to apply heat energy to the tissues and is particularly useful for softening the skin and for relief from muscular and joint pain.

Paraffin wax is a petroleum-based, waxy mixture and conforms well to the shapes of hands, wrists, elbows, knees, ankles and feet.

> **KEY NOTE** Avoid this treatment if there is any acute inflammation, any areas of sensory impairment, any skin disorders or any bruising or swelling. Minor cuts and abrasions may be covered with a waterproof plaster. This treatment is best avoided in very hairy areas.

Method

1. Check the client for contra-indications.
2. Check that the client has removed all jewellery.
3. Cover the floor and treatment couch with a polythene sheet.
4. Check the client's skin is clean.
5. Explain the procedure to the client.

6. Uncover the areas to be treated and protect surrounding areas.
7. Test the temperature of the wax on yourself and on the client (wax should be at working temperature of approximately 49 °C).
8. Pain the wax on to the areas to be treated with a wide brush, working quickly and covering the areas with several layers of wax. The back, legs, feet, hands and arms may be treated in this way.
9. Wrap the treated area in a polythene sheet, grease proof paper or tin foil and then add a towel or warm covering.
10. Leave the client to rest for approximately 15 to 20 minutes.
11. Unwrap the client and ensure that all the wax is removed from the skin. The wax can be lifted off the skin, or will slide away. Pat the area dry.
12. Dispose of used wax into the bin.
13. Proceed with massage treatment (see page 95).

Infra-red Light

Infra-red rays are electromagnetic waves with wavelengths of between 700 nm and 400,000 nm. The two types of lamps that produce infra-red rays are the non-luminous, infra-red lamp, and the more commonly used non-luminous, radiant heat lamp.

Infra-red radiation is particularly useful prior to massage as it helps to promote relaxation. It helps to increase the circulation in preparation for treatment and provides relief from pain and tension.

> **KEY NOTE** Avoid infra-red treatment in areas of sensory impairment, cases of skin diseases and disorders, fever, hypersensitivity, migraine and headaches, blood pressure disorders, heart conditions, diabetes, thrombosis or phlebitis, recent scar tissue, recent bruising, haemorrhaging, recent injury and during pregnancy.

Method

1. Check the client for contra-indications.
2. Check the client has removed all jewellery.
3. Clean the skin with cologne to remove sebum.
4. Check that the lamp is in good working order (check there are no dents in the reflector, check leads and that the stand is stable).
5. Position the client comfortably on the couch and cover the areas not being treated.
6. Explain the procedure to the client.
7. Carry out a hot and cold sensitivity test on the client to check for defective sensation.

> **KEY NOTE** To carry out a hot and cold sensitivity test, use two test tubes (one containing hot water and one cold). Ask the client to close their eyes. Touch the areas to be treated gently and randomly with the tubes. Ask the client to identify which tube is which.

8. Protect the client's face, hair and eyes (offer head covering and goggles).
9. Warn the client not to move nearer to or to touch the lamp.
10. When you switch the lamp on, point it away from the client and towards the floor.
11. Position the lamp so that the lamp is parallel with the part to be treated and so that the rays strike at a 90° angle for maximum penetration.
12. **Do Not** position the lamp directly over the client. Select an appropriate distance of between 45–90 cm (18–36 inches) – a good average is 60 cm (24 inches)
13. Remember that the distance of the lamp will be dependent on the client's tolerance and the intensity of the lamp (some have adjustable dials)
14. Treatment timings is usually between 15–30 minutes depending on the client's needs and tolerance level.
15. Ensure that the client is observed closely throughout the treatment.
16. Treatment may be followed by massage (see page 95).

Audio-sonic

These waves are produced by a hand-held applicator which contains an electromagnet. As the head of the appliance is placed on the tissues, a coil moves forwards and backwards, creating an alternate compression and decompression of the tissues.

Audio-sonic treatment has a gentler action than a mechanical vibrator, as it penetrates more deeply into the tissues and is less stimulating on the surface of the skin. Treatment with audio-sonic is indicated particularly for those sensitive areas which may be too painful for deeper manual massage. It is most useful for aiding relaxation of muscle fibres and is particularly effective for relieving tension nodules.

> **KEY NOTE** Avoid using the audio-sonic vibrator over very bony areas and over any inflammatory disorder.

Method

1. Check the client for contra-indications.
2. Check client has removed all jewellery.
3. Position the client in a comfortable and well-supported position.
4. Explain the procedure to the client.
5. Cleanse the skin in the area to be treated.
6. Apply a suitable medium to the area to be treated (talc or oil for normal skins and cream for dry skin).
7. Switch the vibrator on away from the client and test on the back of the hand.
8. Commence the treatment by using the vibrator over the area to be treated in straight lines or in a circular motion, avoiding bony areas.
9. The applicator may be used indirectly on sensitive or bony areas if the therapist places their hand between the client's skin and the vibrator head.
10. Skin reaction and client tolerance will determine treatment timing: treatment timing is

usually between 5 and 15 minutes (treatment should stop when an even erythema is produced).

11. Remove any excess medium.
12. To maintain hygiene, the applicator may be removed and disinfected with surgical wipes.
13. Proceed with manual massage, if appropriate.

Heat-inducing Products

There are other products which may be used prior to massage, such as heat packs which are useful for pain relief. Care should be taken when using hot packs to ensure that insulating materials is placed between the pack and the client's skin.

> **KEY NOTE** It is very important when using any form of heat therapy to refer to the manufacturer's instructions. Ensure that any electrical equipment is checked for safety by a qualified electrician at least once a year. This is a requirement under health and safety legislation.

MASSAGE TECHNIQUES

In general massage techniques are classified into five main categories, which have all developed from the Swedish system:

- effleurage
- petrissage
- frictions
- tapotement
- vibrations.

Effleurage

This is an introductory stroke in massage and is the most frequently used technique. The term 'effleurage' comes from the French word *effleurer* which means to flow or glide.

Technique

The effleurage stroke is a smooth, gliding and flowing stroke that follows the contours of the client's body. It is performed with the palmar surface of the hand, as if the therapist's hands are moulded to the client's body. Both hands may work simultaneously on larger body parts and one hand, thumbs or fingers may work best on smaller areas.

Effleurage is applied effectively by using the walk standing posture, bending the front knee as the movement progresses in order to lean with the body weight and to push down and away. More pressure may be applied by changing the body position to use more body weight.

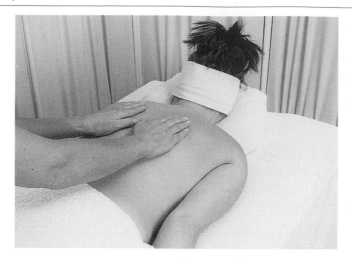

Figure 5.3 Effleurage

Effleurage strokes follow the venous and lymphatic flow. At the end of each stroke, the hands glide back to the starting point with no pressure, ensuring that contact is unbroken. In order to apply effleurage effectively, the therapist's wrist must be flexible and the hands relaxed. Effleurage may either be applied superficially or deeply and is usually applied slowly.

> **KEY NOTE** When applying effleurage, ensure that the angle of the wrist is between 100° and 180° as hyperextension of the wrist may lead to repetitive strain injuries. The therapist's hands, arms, shoulders, back and legs should be aligned along the pathway of the movement.

Benefits and Effects of Effleurage

Effleurage can:

- introduce the client to the therapist's touch
- provide continuity and flow during a massage, by providing the link between other manipulations
- help spread the massage lubricant
- induce a state of relaxation
- warm the tissues, helping to prepare them for deeper strokes
- enhance the effects of other movements and help to remove waste products broken down by deeper manipulations
- soothe areas that are too sore or painful for deeper work
- aid desquamation
- deep effleurage facilitates blood and lymph flow, helping to increase circulation.

Petrissage

The word petrissage comes from the French word *petrir* meaning to knead. In a Swedish massage, petrissage typically follows effleurage. Petrissage incorporates varying manipulations such as palmar kneading, thumb or finger kneading, picking up, wringing and skin rolling. Petrissage has a deeper effect on the circulation than effleurage and helps to address underlying tension in the tissues.

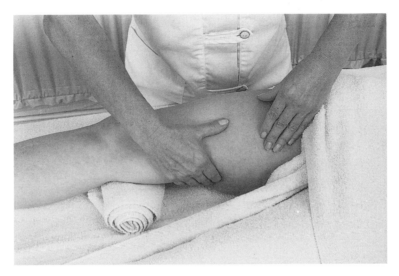

Figure 5.4 Petrissage – palmar kneading

Technique

The application of petrissage is more focused and less generalised than effleurage. It is performed on the fleshy areas of the body. Depending on the area being massaged, petrissage may be applied with one hand or by using both hands alternately. For smaller areas, kneading may be achieved by using the fingers and thumbs.

The basic petrissage technique of kneading involves gently lifting the muscles away from the underlying bones with one hand, holding firmly and squeezing gently the tissues before pressing down to release the tissue into the other hand. In general, pressure should be applied in a rhythmic, circular pattern to achieve alternate compression and relaxation of the muscles. Pressure should be applied smoothly and firmly and then relaxed; hands glide onto an adjacent area and the movement is repeated.

> **KEY NOTE** Rate and rhythm is particularly important with this movement and care should be taken to avoid pinching the skin. It is important to repeat effleurage strokes following petrissage in order to flush out the waste products from the area being worked on.

Benefits and Effects of Petrissage

- Compression and relaxation of the muscle tissue causes the blood and lymphatic vessels to be emptied and filled, thereby increasing circulation and hastening the removal of waste products.
- An improved blood supply accelerates the release of toxins and waste products, such as lactic acid and carbon dioxide, thereby helping to relieve muscle fatigue, soreness and stiffness.
- Petrissage improves cellular nutrition due to an increase in blood supply to the tissues.
- It stretches and broadens the muscle tissue through the action of lifting the muscle away from the bone.
- It relaxes hard, contracted muscles, helping to prevent fibrositis.
- Compression movements can help to maintain the tone and elasticity of muscle tissues, due to an increased blood supply to the muscle.
- Petrissage softens the superficial fascia and can help to loosen adhesions.

Frictions

The term friction comes from the Latin word *frictio*, meaning to rub. Friction typically follows petrissage in a Swedish massage. It is a heat-producing compression stroke which may be performed either superficially to the skin or deeper into the tissue layers of the muscle, using the hands, fingers or thumbs.

Technique

Frictions may be applied in many ways, but in all cases hands, fingers or thumbs should move with the skin's surface so that the underside of the client's skin moves firmly against the underlying muscle, bone or tissue.

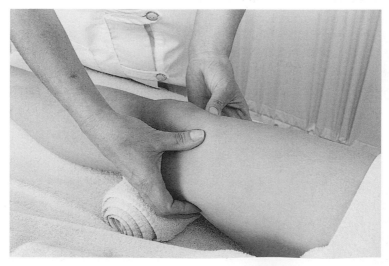

Figure 5.5 Frictions – circular thumb

Frictions may be performed either in a circular or transverse direction. One of the most common types of friction stroke is **circular friction**, in which superficial tissue is moved over deeper tissue. Circular frictions involve the use of the pad of the thumb or fingertips and are concentrated movements, exerting controlled pressure on a small area of tissue and moving it over the underlying structures.

Cross fibre frictions involve the fingers or thumbs moving the skin and fascia back and forth across a muscle, perpendicular to the muscle fibres. It is important to start gently with this technique and gradually progress deeper across the muscle, isolating the stroke to a single muscle or stiff area. As the fingers or thumbs press tissue against tissue, the friction between the fascia and the underlying muscle will warm the area, stretch and soften the fascia, loosen the muscle and break up any adhesions and fibrosis.

> **KEY NOTE** When applying frictions, it is important to move the skin and superficial structures against the deeper structures, without movement taking place on the surface of the skin.
>
> Avoid unnecessary discomfort with this manipulation and intersperse freely with effleurage strokes.

Benefits and Effects of Frictions

Frictions can:

- generate heat
- dilate the capillaries and increase the circulation
- soften and stretch the fascia
- help to break down and separate adhered tissue, freeing restricted areas and tightness
- help to prevent the formation of fibrosis in the tissues
- promotes movement of interstitial fluid between cells and blood vessels
- helps in the absorption of fluid around joints
- have an invigorating effect through the stimulation of nerves.

Tapotement

The word tapotement is derived from the French verb *tapoter*, which means to pat or tap. Tapotement involves a series of percussion movements – quick striking movements – applied to stimulate and activate the underlying tissues.

When applying tapotement it is important to begin with a slow and soft strike, gradually building up to a more forceful stroke. Tapotement is applied rhythmically with either one or two hands. Hands should be flexible and relaxed in order to strike the tissues and spring back after contact. This technique works well on any area with sufficient tissue density and where organ function is safely protected but indirectly stimulated, such as the buttocks, thighs and the upper or mid back.

> **KEY NOTE** Avoid the use of tapotement over vital organs such as the heart, stomach, kidneys and liver and delicate unprotected areas. Tapotement should not be used after exercise as it activates the muscle spindles and may stimulate cramp.

The variations of tapotement technique are **hacking**, **cupping**, **beating** and **pounding**.

Technique for Hacking

This is a light, fast movement performed with the elbows bent and arms abducted. Wrists are extended but hands and fingers should be apart, fairly relaxed and flexed. Hands twist and flick against the skin in rapid succession to produce light glancing movements which strike the body part being treated.

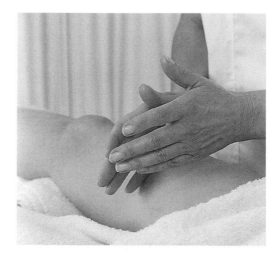

Figure 5.6 Tapotement – hacking

Technique for Cupping

Cupping is performed with the palmar surfaces of the hands, which are formed into loose cups to produce a vacuum-like effect. The cupped hands rhythmically strike the body, producing a distinctive hollow sound. Hands should be cupped loosely and wrists should be relaxed in order that hands bounce quickly and lightly off the skin. It is important to keep hands cupped in order to avoid slapping.

Technique for Beating

This is a heavier manipulation in which the hands form loose fists – the dorsal part of the fingers strike the body and the heel of the hand comes into contact with the area being treated. Beating is delivered rhythmically with alternate hands using moderate pressure. Wrists should be kept loose in order that the fists bounce against the tissues. A change in skin colour and temperature should be instantaneous if this movement is applied correctly.

Technique for Pounding

This is another form of heavy tapotement in which the hands are formed into fists and the outer border of the hands are used to accomplish the movements. The loosely clenched fists strike the tissues and turn inwards back towards the therapist, with each fist circling one another. This technique is performed rapidly and the impetus of the movement comes from the therapist's elbows and forearms.

Benefits and Effects of Tapotement

Tapotement can:

- have a stimulating effect on the circulatory system, increasing local blood flow and erythema
- have a stimulating effect on the nervous system; initially, sensory nerve endings are stimulated to produce an invigorating feeling; the effect becomes sedative if continued
- effect a rise in local skin temperature and metabolism
- help to improve and maintain muscle tone, due to the increased blood flow to the muscles
- help relieve congestion from the chest and back
- help to relieve pain.

Vibrations

These are fine, shaking, trembling or oscillating movements that are applied with one or both hands, using either the whole palmar surface of the hand or the fingertips. A fine, trembling action may be achieved by moving the fingers up and down or from side to side whilst maintaining contact with the skin.

Vibrations may be performed statically or so that the hands or fingertips travel over a point whilst still vibrating. Vibration movements may be fine, deep or vigorous depending on the effect required. Performing vibrations correctly involves co-ordination and practice.

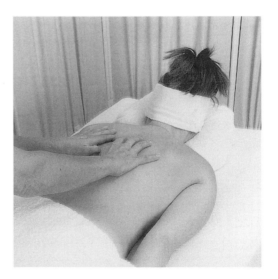

Figure 5.7 Vibrations

Benefits and Effects of Vibrations

Vibrations can:

- help to relieve tension and aid relaxation, having a sedative effect
- stimulate and clear nerve pathways, producing a refreshing effect
- stimulate muscle spindles, thereby creating minute muscle contractions
- help to relieve pain
- help to relieve flatulence if performed over the abdomen.

THERAPEUTIC MASSAGE PROCEDURE

A full body massage will typically include massage to the back, neck, shoulders, chest, legs, feet, hands, arms and abdomen. In a commercial situation, a full body massage will take approximately 1 hour, depending on the needs of the client. Body part massages, such as back, neck and shoulders generally take between 25 and 30 minutes. For practical reasons clients may be unable to have a full body massage and massage may be given locally to a specific area.

> **KEY NOTE** There are many ways of practising therapeutic massage therapy and therapists may differ in their application of movements and the order in which the treatment is given. Experienced massage therapists become instinctive in their touch and can adapt massage techniques to suit the requirements of an individual client.
>
> Whatever techniques are employed and however the techniques are utilised, the common link is that a variety of techniques are used, which are continuous in flow, smooth in rhythm, pressure is adjusted to suit the tissue density, the client's preference and to suit the client's individual needs.

Assessing the tissues

- **Tension** – this may be felt as a tightness in an area of a muscle, as if it is being contracted. Tension in a muscle may be caused by physical or emotional stress. It is important for a therapist to be able to distinguish tense muscles from those which are well toned.

> **KEY NOTE** When massaging a tense muscle, it is important to spend time relaxing the client with effleurage before proceeding to manipulate the tissues to release the tension.

- **Adhesions** – these are abnormal connections between tissues. For example muscles can become stuck together with connective tissue. They are caused by injury, stress or misuse.

> **KEY NOTE** Massage techniques, in particular deep frictions, can help to break adhesions apart and restore normal function to muscles and connective tissue.

- **Fibrosis** – this is a process in which the original type of tissue is replaced by fibrous outer tissue or scar formation. Fibrosis occurs when the damage is such that there are not enough healthy cells to regenerate the tissue required, or when the damaged tissue does not have the ability to reproduce itself. The scar tissue formed by fibrosis is usually stronger than the original tissue.

> **KEY NOTE** Massage can help to restructure the scar tissue formed by fibrosis. By using techniques such as cross fibre frictions the therapist can increase the pliability of the scar tissue and break down adhesions to the surrounding areas.

Adaptations to Massage Procedure

Massage techniques should always be adapted and varied to suit different clients. Differences in physical characteristics, such as body size, muscle tone and age, demand different treatment.

A *standard* massage routine is designed to meet the needs of an *average* client. Throughout their careers, massage therapists encounter many different individuals who require a degree of adaptation due to their physical and health-related situations. Some common client types requiring special treatment are discussed below.

> **KEY NOTE** The best approach to massage is to see every client's situation as a different challenge and to view their individual needs as part of the treatment plan. When adapting a massage, it is not the massage movements that change, the difference is the way in which the therapist modifies or adjust the pressure, speed, duration and frequency of the massage, as well as how the client is positioned.

Adaptations for a Pregnant Client

With a pregnant client the first consideration is to avoid any massage in the first trimester, until the pregnancy is established. If the client has a history of miscarriage or there are complications with the pregnancy everything, including massage, may be suspected should there be a problem.

The second consideration when massaging a pregnant client is comfortable positioning. It is important for the therapist to discuss the best positioning with the client for ease of comfort. During the second and third trimester the client may receive massage in the supine position, lying on one side or, if heavily pregnant, sitting in a chair. Care should be taken to provide plenty of support for the chest and lower abdominal area, and ankles and knees. If ankles are swollen, it is helpful to elevate the knees and the feet using bolsters while supine. The feet should be higher than the knees.

Deep abdominal massage should be avoided during pregnancy, and pressure strokes in general should be soothing and relaxing.

Adaptations for a Disabled Client

The therapist must establish the nature of the disability and, if necessary, research the condition before the consultation. It is important for the therapist to enquire tactfully about the limitations of the condition. It is important not to make assumptions just because a client is disabled it does not mean that they are paralysed. If the client uses a wheelchair, the therapist can sit or kneel in order that they may talk eye to eye.

Depending on the client's condition, positioning may be varied and client comfort should always be the main concern. If it is practical within the limitations of the client's physical condition, treatment may be offered on the couch, which may need to be of variable height. If this is not possible, the client may be treated whilst sitting in their wheelchair; in this case provide plenty of pillows and support so that the client can lean on the treatment couch.

It is essential not to appear patronising, as many disabled clients are very fit and able. They should not be discriminated against because of their disability.

Adaptations for an Elderly Client
There are several considerations to be borne in mind when treating an elderly client.
- Take care to ensure that the client is warm enough throughout the treatment; have extra coverings available.
- Many elderly people experience a sudden drop in blood pressure from time to time. Help the client up to avoid falls.
- Avoid deep massage due to decreased reaction time, possible insensitivity to pain and thinning of skin and blood vessels.
- There may be loss of hearing and vision.
- There will be a decrease in muscle tone and bones may not be strong and flexible; joints may be worn.
- Skin may appear pale, wrinkled, become thinner, looser and more frail.
- The circulation may not be efficient, especially if the client is inactive.

It is best to make the massage sessions short as the client may tire easily.

> **KEY NOTE** Take care when applying pressure and avoid extreme joint mobilisation due to loss of bone integrity.

Adaptations for a Large Client
An important consideration in massaging a large client is the physiological approach to massage. Fatty or adipose tissue presents a different challenge, as muscle tone cannot be assessed easily under a layer of fatty tissue. Pressure should be applied carefully to areas with dense adipose tissue in order to avoid tissue damage and client discomfort. Areas of fatty tissue are not insensitive and care should be taken not to apply too firm a pressure. Adipose tissue is, in fact, highly vascular, making it susceptible to bruising and damage. As with all clients, consider pressure, monitor client feedback and use body mechanics correctly.

The therapist may have to adjust the couch height depending on the size of the client. A client with large breasts may find it more comfortable to use a pillow or some support, either in between the breasts supporting the sternum and chest, or above and below the chest wall when lying prone.

Adaptations for a Thin Client

With a thin client, avoid deep massage or pressure over bony areas which may cause discomfort. Techniques such as tapotement should not be used over unprotected areas. Pressure must be applied carefully and monitored in line with client feedback. However, it is important that the therapist does not assume that a thin client requires a light massage.

Adaptations for a Male Client

In general terms, the male body presents more muscle bulk than the female body and, therefore, an adaptation of technique is required. Male clients generally require a firmer pressure and the therapist should take care to apply the correct body mechanics and posture in order to be able to carry out the techniques effectively and to the client's satisfaction.

If a male client is particularly hairy, use sufficient medium so as not to drag the skin and avoid pulling on the hairs.

With a particularly large male client who has dense tissue bulk, it may be appropriate for the therapist to use adaptations of techniques, such as using the fists to apply petrissage, as opposed to the fingers and thumbs.

Adaptations for Variations in Muscle Tone

Muscles tone may vary due to the physical characteristics of the client and their level of physical activity. Muscle tone is the state of continuous, practical contraction of a muscle in order to maintain body posture. The worst two things for the muscular system are overuse and underuse.

- **Good muscle tone** – the muscles appear firm and rounded. Regular massage will help to keep muscles in good tone. It is more difficult for therapists to massage muscles with good tone as they are firm and less pliable. An adaptation of technique may be needed in order to be able to manipulate the tissues (use more deep effleurage to relax the fascia and tendons).
- **Poor muscle tone** – the muscles appear loose and flattened, rather than rounded. Poor muscle tone may be due to lack of use and lack of regular exercise. Care should be taken when massaging a client with poor muscle tone. Ensure that muscles are not compressed too hard against the underlying bone and that they are not overstreched. Massage may help to increase tone if it is combined with a suitable exercise programme.
- **Muscular atrophy** – this is the wasting away of muscles due to poor nutrition, lack of use or a dysfunction of the motor nerve impulses. Regular use of massage may help to slow down the muscle atrophy; mobilisation of joints and range of motion exercise may also be helpful to encourage movement.
- **Hypertrophy** – this is an increase in the size and diameter of muscle fibres and is usually caused by exercise and weight lifting. Certain manipulations may be more difficult due to the tightness of the muscles. In general, deep effleurage will be helpful for relaxing the muscle fibres and fascia which may have become overstretched.
- **Muscle fatigue** – this is a loss of the ability of a muscle to contract efficiently, due to insufficient oxygen, exhaustion of the energy supply and an accumulation of lactic

acid. Muscle fatigue will cause the muscles to ache; massage strokes such as effleurage and petrissage are useful techniques for eliminating lactic acid.

- **Muscle spasm** – this is an increase in muscle tension due to excessive motor nerve activity, resulting in a knot in the muscle. Muscle spasms cannot be released by voluntary relaxation. However, massage can be a useful aid to relax the muscle fibres.
- **Muscle cramp** – this is an acute, painful contraction of a single muscle or group of muscles. Cramp is often associated with a mineral deficiency, an irritated nerve or muscle fatigue. Cramp may be relieved by pushing firmly and together the belly of the muscle or by stretching out the affected muscles. The muscle should be lengthened after the cramp has subsided.
- **Spasticity** – this is characterised by an increase in muscle tone and stiffness. In severe cases, movement may become unco-ordinated. Spasticity muscles have excessive tone, and are often associated with nervous dysfunction. Use massage techniques that relax the muscle fibres (effleurage and gentle petrissage), taking care to avoid manipulations that are too stimulating on the nervous system.

REACTIONS TO MASSAGE THERAPY

It is important for therapists to understand that a reaction to massage is a positive indication that healing is taking place. The release of unwanted toxins may cause temporary feelings of discomfort until a sense of balance has been restored. It should be stressed to clients that reactions are transitory and that they are part of the body's natural healing process.

Typical reactions to massage therapy include:
- **Aching and soreness of the muscles** – due to the release of toxins it is not unusual for clients to feel as though their muscles have been worked the day after treatment, particularly if deep massage has been carried out. The best piece of advice to give a client is to drink plenty of water and to avoid overexerting the body while the healing process is taking place.
- **Tiredness** – clients may experience tiredness due to the flood of toxins being released into the bloodstream and to the utilisation of energy by the body for repair. Clients should be advised, therefore, to take a suitable rest period.
- **Renewed energy** – some clients may feel very energetic and revitalised following massage, due to the release of toxins. Clients should be advised to avoid tapping into this energy too soon as they may over exert themselves.
- **Emotional release** – occasionally clients may feel emotional due to the release of repressed tension. This release should be encouraged and seen as a positive sign.
- **Dizziness** – Clients who get up too quickly may feel dizzy or faint due to a drop in blood pressure, especially if the body has been in a state of deep relaxation.

Contra-actions to Massage Therapy

A contra-action to massage is a reaction that may occur either during or after the massage treatment. It is important that therapists are able to identify a contra-action, and are aware of what to do in the event of one occurring.

Skin Reactions

Therapists should monitor the client's skin tolerance to the massage medium, and if the client has a sensitive skin it is advisable to carry out a patch test (see page 78). With a sensitive skin, the medium is chosen carefully, avoiding any perfumes or any sensitising ingredients.

If the client develops a skin reaction to the oil or lotion, the skin will become blotchy, inflamed and red. If a skin reaction occurs, the product should be removed with warm water as soon as possible and then the skin should be left alone. If the reaction continues, the client should seek medical advice. In the case of clients with allergies to nuts, avoid oils which are but-based.

Erythema

Massage stimulates tissue to release histamines and acetylcholine. The release of these chemicals causes erythema which is an observable reddening of the skin that results from increased blood flow.

This reddening or flushing of the skin may be a physiological sign that the massage is reaching the deeper layers of the skin, increasing nutrition of the tissues and encouraging removal of waste, or it may be a sign of inflammation or allergy.

> **KEY NOTE** Therapists should take care to record all contra-actions as they occur, along with their effects and any advice given to the client.

HOW THE EFFECTIVENESS OF THE MASSAGE MAY BE JUDGED

In order to assess whether the client's needs are being met, it is helpful to receive some form of feedback from the client during and after the massage.

Feedback may be:
- **Verbal** – the client may indicate their satisfaction verbally throughout or after the massage. If the client books another appointment, this is a good indicator of client satisfaction.
- **Non-Verbal or visual** – the therapist may assess a client's body language and their facial expressions to gain feedback about the success of the treatment.
- **Written** – the client may be asked for their written comments on how the massage felt and whether their needs were met by the treatment.

AFTER CARE ADVICE

Massage unlocks toxins and releases stress and tension held within the soft tissues of the body. Due to the fact that the body experiences heightened toxicity after a massage, clients should be given the following advice:

- **Drink water** – clients should be advised to drink plenty of fresh water to assist the flushing out of any toxins and waste products.
- **Eat a light diet** – the client's diet should be as light as possible after a massage, as the body needs to concentrate its efforts on detoxification and natural healing.
- **Avoid alcohol and smoking** – due to increase in toxins circulating in the body, alcohol and smoking should be avoided.
- **Have a suitable rest period** – clients should be advised to rest as much as possible after a massage in order to assist the healing process and to benefit from the effects of relaxation and stress reduction.
- **Have regular treatments** – clients should be encouraged to book regular massage treatments in order that they may benefit from its positive effects. Having regular treatments can help a client to maintain their physical and emotional well-being.

Home Care Treatment

Clients may be advised on how they can prolong the effects of the massage at home. Suitable home care products which may be retailed to a client include:

- **Massage oils** – which may be used for self-massage and to help improve the condition of the skin.
- **Bath oils** – to prolong the effects of the massage and help with relaxation and stress relief at home.
- **Massage mitts** – these are designed to stimulate a sluggish circulation and remove dead skin cells.
- **Moisturisers** – the regular use of a body moisturiser massaged into the skin will help to hydrate the skin.
- **Mechanical massager** – these are designed to stimulate the effects of a manual massage and may be a useful back up to treatments with a therapist.

CHAPTER 6

Aromatherapy massage

INTRODUCTION

Aromatherapy is defined as the systematic use of essential oils in holistic treatments to help improve physical and emotional well-being. Aromatherapy is a truly holistic therapy in that it aims to treat the whole person by taking account, not only of their physical state but also their emotions. Emotions can have a profound effect on general well-being.

Aromatherapy is a term that encompasses many forms of treatment. However, this chapter is devoted to aromatherapy treatment via massage.

BRIEF HISTORY AND DEVELOPMENT OF AROMATHERAPY

The first evidence of wide-ranging use of aromatic oils comes from the ancient Egyptians who, as far back as 3000 BC, extracted oils by a method of infusion. They used these extracts in a wide variety of ways: as cosmetics, for religious ceremonies, in massage, surgery, food preservation and for mummification. Records in the Bible from around 2000 BC show the use of plants and aromatic oils in the treatment of illness and in religious ceremonies. Ancient Chinese pharmacopoeia (medical texts) list herbs with scents that were thought to have therapeutic effects. Ancient Hindu scriptures list hundred of aromatic substances for religious and therapeutic use.

From China, India and Egypt the art of aromatherapy spread to Ancient Greece and Rome where the oils were used for aromatic massages and in daily baths. Hippocrates, the Greek physician, advocated the use of aromatic oils and wrote about a vast range of medicinal plants claiming that the best way to achieve good health was to have an aromatic bath and scented massage every day. Hippocrates' writings were translated into Arabic languages. The most famous Arab physician was Avicenna who is credited with inventing the refrigerated coil, a development of a more primitive form of distillation, which was used to produce pure oil and aromatic waters.

The earliest written record of the use of aromatic oils in Europe was in the thirteenth century. However, essential oil production was not widely practised until the sixteenth century. Between 1470–1670 there was a proliferation of publications called 'herbals'. These were books about the medicinal properties of plants. Nicholas Culpeper, a celebrated herbalist, wrote *A Book of Herbs* in 1652 which contained the medicinal properties of hundreds of plants. The medicinal properties of the oils were verified by the fact that those people using them during this period were the ones to survive the plague that struck Europe.

The scientific study of the therapeutic properties of essential oils was commenced by the French cosmetic chemist Gattefosse in the 1920s. He discovered, after burning his arm in a laboratory, that the essential oil of lavender was exceptionally healing on the skin and left no scarring. Other French doctors and scientists continued his work, most notably Dr Jean Valnet. He used essential oils to treat burns and battle injuries, in the absence of medical supplies.

Despite research to validate essential oils as scientifically proven substances, essential oils started to lose credibility. This was due to the growth of the modern synthetic drug industry. The use of essential oils was reduced to being included in perfumes and cosmetics, and use as food flavourings.

Aromatherapy was re-introduced into Britain in the 1950s by Marguerite Maury, who was a student of Dr Gattefosse. She developed Gattefosse's work on a more practical level by combining the use of essential oils with massage. She developed specialised aromatherapy massage techniques and proposed the holistic approach of the '**individual prescription**', selecting and blending oils to suit the individual needs of the client. The techniques that Marguerite Maury introduced into Britain are those which underpin the practice of aromatherapy today.

Despite its ancient origins, aromatherapy is still in its clinical infancy. More research and extensive clinical practice are being carried out to validate the effects of essential oils on the mind and body. Today, it is one of the most popular and fast growing complementary therapies.

HOW AROMATHERAPY WORKS

There are two ways in which essential oils may be absorbed into the bloodstream for therapeutic effect; **through the skin** and **via respiration**. There is some degree of debate as to whether essential oils work because of their chemical constituents or because of their route of administration, massage for example.

However, it is generally accepted that the effects of aromatherapy upon the body are diverse because essential oils have three distinct modes of action:

1. They initiate chemical changes in the body when the essential oil enters the bloodstream and reacts with hormones and enzymes.
2. They have physiological effects on the systems of the body.
3. They have psychological effects when the odour of the oil is inhaled.

The Absorption of Essential Oils into the Bloodstream
The Skin

Essential oils are absorbed into the body via the skin by simple diffusion. Absorption is assisted by the fact that the skin is semi-permeable and the aromatic molecules of essential oils are fat-soluble. Essential oil molecules, therefore, dissolve in the sebum produced by the sebaceous glands and pass into the dermis via the micro-circulation (capillaries). They are carried by the blood and lymphatic system and are transported throughout the body.

The rate of absorption of essential oils may be dependent on several factors:
- the composition of the oil (oils with a lower volatility take longer to absorb)
- the viscosity of the carrier oil or oils
- the condition of the client's skin (excess fat, oedema, sluggish circulation and excess tissue toxication will slow down absorption).

Factors that can enhance the absorption of essential oils include:
- stimulation and increased blood flow (via massage)

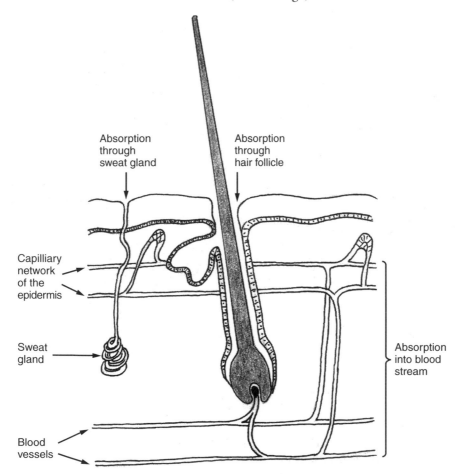

Figure 6.1 The absorption of essential oils into the skin

- heat (the treatment room should be comfortably warm; clients should be covered during and kept warm after the massage in order to aid absorption)
- clean skin – ideally clients should come for treatment pre-showered with all body creams and lotions removed
- the client may also be encouraged to carry out dry skin brushing prior to an aromatherapy massage in order to remove the dead keratinised layer of the skin.

> **KEY NOTE** The amount of essential oil molecules reaching the bloodstream will be greatly enhanced if the client is encouraged to breathe deeply throughout an aromatherapy massage.

Elimination of Essential Oils from the Bloodstream

Essential oils are eliminated from the body in different ways:

- through the renal system in urine
- through the skin in sweat
- through the intestines in faeces
- through the respiratory system in exhaled breath.

The Physiology of Respiration

The respiratory system plays an important part in an aromatherapy massage treatment. The fine, volatile, essential oil molecules are carried into the lungs with the inspired air and are absorbed into the bloodstream. Being volatile means that liquid oil molecules easily become gas. It is gaseous molecules that are breathed in.

Once the molecules have entered the respiratory pathway via the nose, the molecules travel into the nasopharynx, pharynx, larynx, trachea and to the lungs via the bronchi. Within the lungs the bronchi divide and subdivide, finally forming bronchioles ending in microscopic air sacs or **alveoli**. This is where gas exchange takes place. Each cluster of alveoli is surrounded by a rich network of capillaries and a moist membrane. The inhaled air, carrying essential oil molecules diffuses through the membrane which is one cell thick. Once in the blood vessels, oxygen and any other molecules carried with it are transported, partially in solution and partially bound to the haemoglobin.

The Theory of Olfaction

Olfaction is the process of odour perception. The process of olfaction may be summarised as follows:

1 Reception

- The volatile molecules of the essential oil evaporate on contact with warm air (some volatile molecules pervade the air and some enter the nose).
- The odiferous molecules of the essential oil dissolve in the mucous which lines the inner nasal cavity.

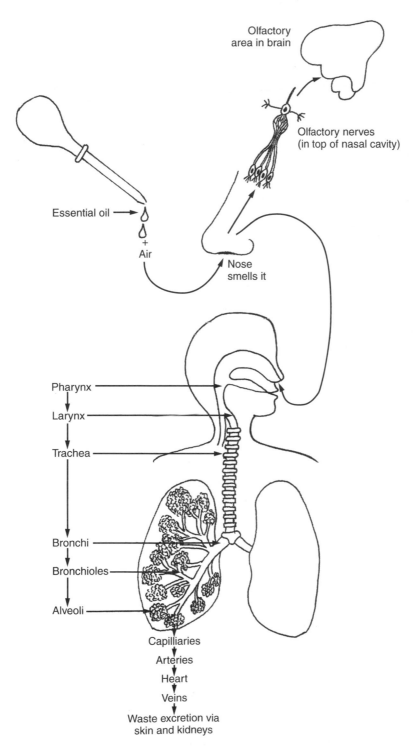

Figure 6.2 The absorption of essential oils via the respiratory system

2 Transmission

■ These aromatic molecules are picked up by the cilia which protrude from the **olfactory receptor cells** (located at the top of the nasal cavity).

■ The olfactory receptor cells have a long nerve fibre, called an **axon**. An electrochemical message of the aroma is transmitted along the axons of receptor cells and is passed on to the **olfactory nerves**.

■ The fibres of the olfactory nerves pass through the cribriform plate of the ethmoid bone in the roof of the nose to reach the **olfactory bulb**. Here the nerve signal is chemically converted before being relayed to the brain.

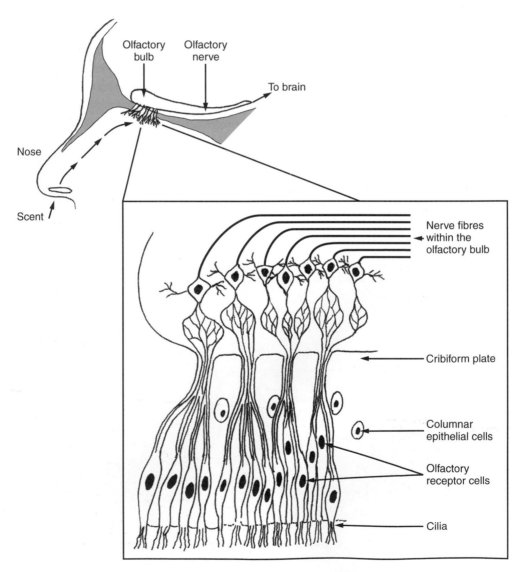

Figure 6.3 The theory of olfaction

3 Perception

- Once the message reaches the olfactory bulb, the olfactory impulses pass into the olfactory tract. From here they travel directly to the cerebral cortex where the smell is perceived.
- The **temporal lobe** of the brain contains the **primary olfactory area**, which is directly connected to the **limbic area**.

> **KEY NOTE** Smell is the only sense that has a direct access route to the brain.

The Limbic Area of the Brain

Originally known as the 'smell brain', the limbic system is a complex ring of brain structures and interconnected pathways. It is situated at the top of the brain stem.

The main parts of the limbic system include:

- **The amalygda** – which is thought to work with the hypothalamus to mediate emotional responses.
- **The hippocampus** – which is the part of the limbic system that helps link an odour to a memory.

So, smell is the sense that connects directly with the limbic system, which houses our emotions, sexual feelings, memory and learning. As the anterior part of the limbic system is in the olfactory cortex this explains the intimate relationship between smells and emotion.

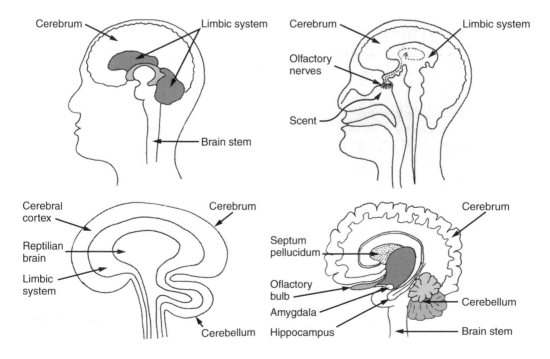

Figure 6.4 The limbic system

The limbic system also has multiple connections with other parts of the brain such as the thalamus, hypothalamus and the pituitary gland. This explains how olfaction can influence endocrine function and help regulate autonomic nervous activity.

> **KEY NOTE** The complexity of the limbic system and the direct link between olfaction and the limbic area of the brain explains how smell can evoke an emotional response in the brain, make us recall a memory from the past and can help to restore a sense of well-being in the body.

BENEFITS AND EFFECTS OF AROMATHERAPY MASSAGE

Due to the diversity of essentials oils and their individual therapeutic properties, the range of benefits and effects of aromatherapy massage is wide ranging.

Physiological Benefits

Aromatherapy massage can:
- enhance lymphatic drainage – this helps to reduce fluid retention and prevent oedema
- induce a feeling of deep relaxation in the body
- help to restore balance in the body
- stimulate the body's natural immune system
- increase the oxygen and nutrient supply to the tissues by increasing the blood circulation
- can help to increase energy levels as blockages and congestion in the nerves are eased.

Psychological Benefits

Aromatherapy massage can:
- promote a general state of well-being
- calm and soothe the mind
- help to reduce nervous tension
- help to lift the mood and reduce feelings of depression.

CAUTIONS AND CONTRA-INDICATIONS FOR AROMATHERAPY MASSAGE

As the benefits of aromatherapy massage are so far reaching, it is tempting to assume it will be beneficial for everyone. However, there are certain precautions that have to be taken and restrictions on treatment, depending on the medical condition of the client at the time of the proposed treatment.

In certain cases it may be necessary to refer the client to their GP before treatment is applied. Where possible, treatment should be adapted to suit the client's conditions and needs.

It should be remembered that clients with medical conditions may present with factors that may increase the effects of the essential oils used (a combination of the client's condition and medication may cause the client to have a more pronounced reaction to the treatment). However, there are many essential oils whose effects may benefit a client's condition. For instance, lavender essential oil, combined with the relaxing effects of an aromatherapy massage, may help to lower a client's blood pressure and to improve their general circulation.

Medical advice should always be sought when treating a client with a medical condition to reduce the risk of adverse effects. The choice of essential oil for a client in this position should be based on common sense and reliable clinical data, if available. Whilst massage may be contra-indicated for certain conditions, other forms of aromatherapy treatment may be suitable (such as inhalation, compresses, skin creams and lotions).

- **Fever** – in the case of a fever, there is a risk of spreading the infection due to the increase in circulation created by a massage. During fever, body temperatures rises as a result of infection.
- **Infectious diseases** (colds, flu, measles, tuberculosis, scarlet fever) – these are contra-indicated due to the fact they are contagious.
- **Skin diseases** – care should be taken to avoid cross infection and spreading the infection.
- **Recent haemorrhage** – haemorrhaging is excessive bleeding which may be either internal or external. Massage should be avoided due to the risk of increasing blood loss from the blood vessels. If in any doubt, medical advice should be sought.
- See also page 119 for conditions that are contra-indicated for massage treatment.
- **Severe circulatory disorders and heart conditions** – medical clearance should be sought. There is a risk that the increase in circulation resulting from the aromatherapy massage may overburden the heart. There may be an increase in the risk of thrombus or embolus. If medical clearance is given, the aromatherapy massage should be applied lightly and gently.

KEY NOTE The use of essential oils such as lavender and marjoram may help a client with a heart condition as they are considered to be heart sedatives.

- **Thrombosis** – medical clearance should be sought. There is a risk that the increased circulation due to the aromatherapy massage may move a clot to the heart. If medical clearance is given, the massage should be applied lightly and gently.
- **High blood pressure** – clients with high blood pressure should have a medical referral prior to aromatherapy massage, even if they are on prescribed medication, due to their susceptibility to form clots. Clients taking anti-hypertensive medication may be prone to postural hypotension and may feel light-headed and dizzy after treatment.

Assist the client off the couch and ensure that they get up slowly. Once medical clearance is given, aromatherapy massage should be soothing and relaxing.

> **KEY NOTE** There are several essential oils which are said to help lower blood pressure. These include clary sage, lavender, lemon, marjoram and sweet orange.

- **Low blood pressure** – a client with low blood pressure may experience dizziness and could fall when sitting or standing after massage.

> **KEY NOTE** Avoid essential oils which are more sedative and help to lower blood pressure, in particular lavender and marjoram.

- **Epilepsy** – medical advice should always be sought prior to massaging a client with a history of epilepsy.

> **KEY NOTE** Avoid the use of oils which are too stimulating or too deeply relaxing to reduce the risk of convulsions. An important consideration is the choice of aroma as some types of epilepsy may be triggered by smells.

- **Diabetes** – clients with diabetes require medical referral as they may be prone to arteriosclerosis, high blood pressure and oedema. Pressure should be carefully monitored during massage as the client may have loss of sensory nerve function. They may be unable to give accurate feedback regarding pressure. If the client is receiving injections, avoid aromatherapy massage on recent injection sites. Clients should have their necessary medication with them when they attend for treatment, in case of an emergency.
- **Cancer** – medical clearance should always be sought before carrying out an aromatherapy treatment on a client who has a cancerous condition. There is a theoretical risk that certain types of cancer may spread through the lymphatic system. Aromatherapy massage may aid in the metasis of the cancer.

Advice should always be sought from the consultant or medical team in charge of the client's care before proceeding. Aromatherapy massage treatment, if advised by the medical team, should be light and short. Usually it is confined to specific areas, such as the hand, face and feet. When massaging a cancer patient, avoid areas of the body which are receiving radiation therapy, are close to tumour sites or are areas of skin cancer.

> **KEY NOTE** It is well known that certain essential oils and gentle aromatherapy massage can be beneficial to cancer patients. This helps with palliative health care by enabling the patient to cope psychologically with their condition and by alleviating some of the side effects of the cancer treatment.

■ **Skin disorders** – some conditions may be exacerbated or worsened by aromatherapy massage. Some inflamed skin conditions should be treated as a localised contra-indication.

KEY NOTE Stress-related skin conditions in particular respond favourably to aromatherapy.

■ **Recent scar tissue** – aromatherapy massage should only be applied to scar tissue once it has fully healed and can withstand pressure.

KEY NOTE The use of essential oils such as lavender, frankincense and neroli can promote healing and cell regeneration.

■ **Severe bruising** – localised massage is contra-indicated in order to avoid discomfort and pain.
■ **Varicose veins** – avoid direct pressure on or around a varicose vein. If severe, medical clearance may be necessary as the client may be prone to thrombosis. Gentle aromatherapy massage given proximally to the areas may help to reduce oedema and prevent venous and lymphatic stasis.
■ **Cuts and abrasions** – these should be avoided as aromatherapy massage could further damage the healing tissue and expose the client and therapist to infection.
■ **Recent fractures and sprains** – it is important to seek medical clearance before massaging a sprain or similar injury due to the increased risk of vascular bleeding.
■ **Undiagnosed lumps, bumps and swellings** – clients should be referred to their GP for a diagnosis. Aromatherapy massage may cause damage in the area by virtue of pressure and motion.

Special Factors to be Taken into Consideration Before an Aromatherapy Massage

■ **Asthma** – the use of specific essential oils with aromatherapy massage may help breathing difficulties such as asthma. Take care to avoid certain essential oils or carrier oils depending on the client's allergies.
■ **Allergies and skin intolerances** – a patch test should be carried out before treatment commences in order to eliminate the risk of adverse reaction to the proposed essential oils.
■ **Medication** – the use of certain essential oils may exacerbate the excretion of drugs by speeding up detoxification in the liver. However, the interaction between essential oils and drugs is an area that remains unexplored and is largely undocumented.

■ **Homeopathic preparations** – there is no proof that aromatherapy interferes with homeopathic treatment. However, some people believe the actions and strong odours of certain essential oils (such as peppermint) may antidote homeopathic treatment. Others feel that aromatherapy may enhance homeopathic treatment. If a client is undergoing homeopathic treatment at the time of an aromatherapy massage, they should consult their homeopath to ensure that the proposed treatment is in synergy with the homeopathic preparations.

■ **Abdominal treatment for women during menstruation** – the abdominal area may be omitted from the aromatherapy massage during menstruation to avoid discomfort. However, some clients may find massaging the lower back helpful in offering pain relief and comfort.

■ **Pregnancy** – as essential oils cross the placental barrier, they have the potential to affect the foetus. It is wise to avoid any form of treatment to a pregnant women during the first trimester of pregnancy. Thereafter, if the pregnancy is uncomplicated, use a lower dilution of oils and research known safety data to avoid potentially toxic essential oils that may be harmful to mother and foetus.

■ **Migraine** – it is felt that some strong or heavy odours may precipitate or exacerbate the effects of a migraine. Careful choice of oils is needed in consultation with the client.

■ **Children and babies** – small people require special care and handling. A lower dilution of oils (1% or less) should be used. Avoid all toxic oils.

KEY NOTE Recommended oils for children include roman chamomile, lavender, rose and gentle citrus oils such as mandarin.

SAFETY PRECAUTIONS

Although essential oils are natural, botanical substances, this does not guarantee their safety. When using essential oils for aromatherapy massage, the following precautions should be observed to ensure a safe and effective treatment, with no adverse effects for either the client or the aromatherapist:

■ Always work in a well ventilated area.

■ Keep and dispense oils away from the treatment area.

■ Air the treatment room in between clients and allow yourself a break in between treatments.

■ Keep essential oils away from the eyes and other sensitive parts of the face.

■ Always carry out a detailed consultation to establish the client's physical and psychological condition, along with any medication they may be taking.

■ Refer clients under medical care to their GP for advice on their suitability for the proposed treatment before proceeding.

■ Never take essential oils by mouth, vagina or rectum, unless under medical instructions.

■ Never apply essential oils to the skin in their undiluted form.

■ Always use essential oils in sensible proportions and follow recommended blending ratios.

■ Avoid prolonged use of the same essential oil.

■ If a client is susceptible to allergies and sensitivity, always carry out a patch test before using the proposed essential oil or oils and record the results.

■ Always label all blends.

■ Only use genuine, authentic essential oils for therapeutic application.

■ Always keep a record of the essential oils blended for each client and their ratios, along with any adverse reactions that may occur.

■ Never use essential oils for where there is no safety data available or with which you are unfamiliar.

Toxicity

Toxicity is a broad term used to describe the hazardous effects associated with the misuse of essential oils. There are two main categories of toxicity:

1. **Acute toxicity** – this refer to the short-term administration of a essential in a high dose. The type of reaction that occurs will depend on the route of administration and the quantities used. There are two types of acute toxicity.

■ **Acute oral toxicity** – this is when an essential oil is taken in a high dose orally, possibly leading to poisoning or death.

■ **Acute dermal toxicity** – this is when high levels of essential oils are applied to the skin. This may result in systemic toxicity and damage to the liver and kidneys.

2. **Chronic toxicity** – this refers to the repeated use of essential oils over a period of weeks, months or years, possibly leading to adverse effects such as headaches, nausea, minor skin eruptions and lethargy.

Types of Unsafe Oils

Toxic Essential Oils

Essential oils known to have high levels of toxicity include:

■ aniseed
■ arnica
■ mugwort
■ pennyroyal
■ sassafras
■ savory
■ thuja
■ wintergreen
■ wormwood.

These oils should be avoided in aromatherapy treatments.

Potentially Carcinogenic Essential Oils

Little is known about the potentially carcinogenic substances found in some essential oils. There is no evidence to suggest that either essential oils or aromatherapy have ever caused cancer. However, essential oils with significant levels of certain compounds are considered to be *potentially* carcinogenic. For safety reasons use of essential oils such as basil (high estragole), camphor brown and yellow and sassafras should be avoided in aromatherapy. It is also advisable that anethole-rich essential oils, such as fennel, should be avoided for those with oestrogen-dependent cancers, such as breast cancer.

> **KEY NOTE** Remember that the majority of essential oils are perfectly harmless. The only cases of poisoning that have been reported are cases of excessive overdose, in some cases 50 to 200 times the recommended dose.

Other Reactions to Essential Oils
Phototoxicity

Phototoxicity refers to a chemical reaction that takes place in the skin, The damage is caused by the combination of a phototoxic oil and ultra-violet rays (from natural or artificial sunlight). Phototoxic reactions range from a mild skin colour change to rapid tanning and hyperpigmentation. Depending on the severity of the reaction, it may cause blistering or deep weeping burns.

> **KEY NOTE** Essential oils which may present a risk of phototoxicity include:
> - bergamot (expressed)
> - lemon (expressed)
> - bitter orange (expressed)
> - lime (expressed)
> - grapefruit (expressed).

Irritation

Irritation is the most common type of skin reaction to essential oil. It is caused when a substance, such as an essential oil, reacts with the mast cells of the skin which release histamine. The term 'irritation' refers to localised inflammation which may affect the skin and mucous membranes. Along with varying degrees of inflammation the skin may itch. Irritation is dose dependent. This means that the reaction is directly proportional to the amount of oil used.

> **KEY NOTE** Essential oils which may present a risk of irritation include:
> - cinnamon leaf
> - clove bud
> - clove stem
> - clove leaf
> - red thyme
> - wild thyme.
>
> Some more common essential oils may also cause irritation if used in excessive proportions, or if used undiluted on the skin.

Sensitisation

Sensitisation is an allergic reaction to an essential oil and involves an inflammatory reaction. This is caused when the cells of the immune system (T-lymphocytes) become sensitised. Following the first exposure to the essential oil, the effects on the skin may be slight; on repeated application of the same substance, the immune system produces a reaction similar to dermal irritation, The skin may appear blotchy and irritated.

KEY NOTE Essential oils which may present a risk of sensitisation include:
- cinnamon (bark, leaf and stem)
- ginger
- lemon
- lemongrass
- lime
- melissa
- bitter orange
- peppermint
- teatree
- thyme.

Safe Handling of Essential Oils

Essential oils are highly concentrated substances and may be hazardous if misused. Great care should be taken when handling them.

Care should be taken by aromatherapists to:
- ensure that, when handling essential oil bottles, their skin does not come into contact with the undiluted oil, and that it is not transferred to more sensitive parts (nose, face and neck for example)
- avoid contact with essential oils if their hands are cracked and sore
- wash hands thoroughly in between clients
- ensure that the correct tops are put back on the correct bottles and that the tops are tightly secured.
- avoid prolonged exposure to essential oils.

KEY NOTE The amount of essential oil absorbed by the therapist during an aromatherapy massage will vary (roughly $\frac{1}{2}$ to 2 drops). Since these quantities are small, the resultant effect on the aromatherapist should be minimal. The skin on the hands is thicker than on other areas of the body. This prevents the essential oils from penetrating into the deeper layers and being absorbed into the bloodstream. Washing hands thoroughly after the massage can help to remove any residual oil. Provided aromatherapists work in a well ventilated room (breathing air saturated with essential oils could be overstimulating) and that regular breaks are taken, they should not suffer the adverse effects of the oils.

Storage of Essential Oils

The following guidelines are recommended for safe storage and to prolong the life of the essential oils:

- Store in dark glass bottles at a normal to cool temperature with lids tightly secured to avoid oxidisation and degradation of the oil.
- Keep in a dark place, away from bright lights.
- Store out of reach of children (some aromatherapists may wish to use childproof caps).
- Keep away from naked flames, as the oils are highly flammable.

Labelling of Essential Oils

All essential oils sold for professional or home use should have safety precautions included in their labelling. The Code of Practice, recommended by the Aromatherapy Trade Council (ATC) – an independent body formed in 1992 by responsible essential oils suppliers – is as follows:

a) Integral, single drop dispensers are to be incorporated in all bottles of essential oil on sale to the general public.

b) The following warnings should be printed on the label:

- Instructions for use (add 5 drops of essential oil to 10 ml of carrier, for instance).
- Keep away from children.
- Keep away from delicate areas such as the eyes.
- Do not apply undiluted to the skin.
- Do not take internally.
- The quantity of essential oil in the bottle.
- The company's name and address.

> **KEY NOTE** The Medicines Act of 1968 clearly states that no medicinal claims can be made on the labels, promotional material or advertisements of products that have not been licensed. This means that no aromatherapy product can make remedial claims relating to a specific disease or condition.

ESSENTIAL OILS

Essential oils are produced in plants during photosynthesis (one of a plant's metabolic processes). They are usually present in minute quantities (making up 0.01 to 10% of the mass of the whole plant).

Essential oils are extracted from various part of aromatic plants: leaves, flowers, fruit, grass, roots, wood, bark, gum and blossom. The essential oil is what gives the plant its fragrance.

As well as being highly concentrated and aromatic, essential oils are also volatile and are immiscible (do not mix) with water.

Essential oils vary in density; most essential oils are liquid, although some, such as Sandalwood, are more viscous. Most essential oils are pale or colourless, but some are more coloured (such as the citrus oils that are expressed from the fruit).

The Chemistry of Essential Oils

Essential oils are made up of basic organic elements: carbon, hydrogen and oxygen. Essential oils may contain as little as 10 or as many as 200 different chemical components. They have a highly complex chemical structure and little is known about the pharmacological actions of all their constituents. This means that essential oils are hard to analyse.

The therapeutic value and potential toxicology of essential oils relate to their chemistry. Each essential oil has it own unique chemical profile and the therapeutic properties are largely determined by the combination and the concentration of its chemical composition.

> **KEY NOTE** It is important to remember that it is virtually impossible to generalise about the therapeutic properties of an essential oil based on the properties of the known chemical constituents alone. By taking such as approach to analysis, you lose sight of the effects of the whole oil.

Methods of Extraction of Essential Oils

Due to their differences in distribution, there are different methods of producing essential oils.

Steam Distillation

This is the oldest and most established method of extracting essential oils. In this method, steam is passed through the plant material. This extracts the volatile, aromatic molecules and carries them through a cooling pipe into a container where separation of the essential oil and the water takes place.

Expression

This process can only be used when the aromatic material can be obtained easily without the use of heat. The method is used solely for the citrus fruits and involves pressing the **essence** from under the surface of the fruit rind.

Solvent Extraction

This process involves using a volatile solvent to extract the odiferous part of the plant. The method is used to extract fragrance materials which do not withstand the heat of distillation, or for plants with a very low yield of fragrance material.

During the process of solvent extraction, a creamy solid called a **concrete** (a combination of plant wax and essential oil) is produced. The final aromatic or perfume product which is extracted from the concrete is known as an **absolute**.

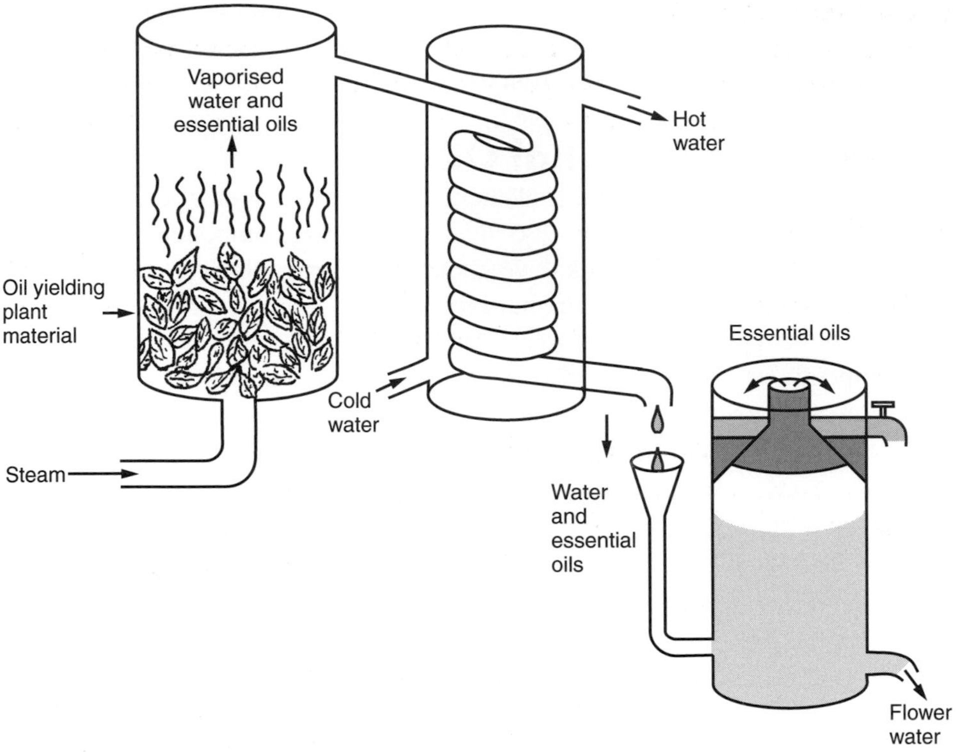

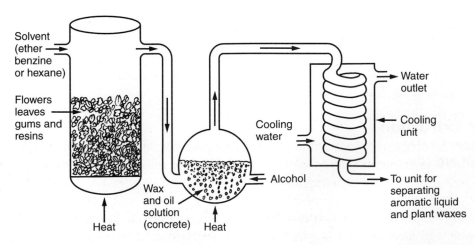

Figure 6.5 Steam distillation

Figure 6.6 Solvent extraction

Carbon Dioxide Extraction

Extraction by liquid carbon dioxide is one method that produces a true smell that is free of any kind of residue carbon dioxide and does not react with the aromatic material during extraction. Extraction by carbon dioxide uses very sophisticated and expensive equipment and, therefore, it is not widely used.

Phytonic Process

This advanced process was developed by Dr Peter Widle in 1987. It is a process that is performed at low temperatures, using the cleanest and most environmentally-friendly technology available. This ensures that the highly fragile and heat sensitive constituents of the essential oil are neither lost nor altered.

Purchasing Quality Essential Oils

In order to purchase quality essential oils it is important to consider the following:

- **Botanical identity and origin** – you should check these to ensure authenticity. There are many species and variations of plants which all exhibit slightly different characteristics. The origin of the plant will determine the essential oil's character and its chemical composition.
- **Cultivation method** – it is useful for an aromatherapist to know how the plant was grown and the environment in which it was cultivated. The plant variety itself, the type of soil and the country of origin will all play a part in determining quality.

> **KEY NOTE** Organic essential oils are those which have been grown in a chemical-free soil. Wild essential oils come from plants which have been grown in their natural habitat, such as at high altitude or in the rainforest.

- **Method of extraction** – it is important not only to ensure that the starting materials used to produce the oil represent the natural biochemistry of the plant, but when it is produced it is of the highest quality.
- **Purity** – a pure essential oil can be defined as one which has been produced from a botanical source and that has not been modified in any that alters it unique qualities. Aromatherapists should ask suppliers for information about the methods used to test for purity. The best advice is to purchase essential oils from a professional supplier who is prepared to pass on as much information as possible: the nature of the oils, their purity, extraction methods and origin.

> **KEY NOTE** A supplier of essential oils may use a method for testing essential oils called **Gas Liquid Chromatography** (GLC). This is a way of determining an oil's chemical composition and will highlight any undesirable substances, such as trace contaminants. Whilst Gas Liquid Chromatography will highlight chemical imbalances in the oil, it is not a guaranteed method of purity.

Shelf Life of Essential Oils

As most essential oils do gradually degrade, it is recommended that they are used within two years of first opening. Citrus oils have a relatively short shelf life and even under good storage conditions, will only remain unchanged for up to a year.

> **KEY NOTE** It is useful to have a 'best before' date on bottles and to monitor the shelf life of essential oils.

Adulteration of Essential Oils

Due to their highly complex chemistry, essential oils are impossible to reproduce exactly by synthetic means. Unfortunately, due to the widespread commercialism in the aromatherapy trade, there is an increase in the practice of adulteration. This involves adding cheaper substitutes to the oil.

Synthetic substances and reconstructed oils have been used successfully in perfumery, as food flavourings and as pharmaceuticals. In aromatherapy, however, it is vital that an essential oil remains in its natural state in order to give the desired therapeutic effects. Adulterated oils may cause skin reactions due to the synthetic additives.

> **KEY NOTE** Essential oils which have been adulterated by redistillation, reconstruction or by the addition of synthetic substances will smell slightly harsher as they do not have the same natural balance of chemicals as the pure oil.

ALPHABETICAL LIST OF ESSENTIAL OILS

Bergamot (Citrus bergamia)

Plants origin: fruit
Method of extraction: expressed
Aroma characteristics: light and delicate lemon or orange aroma with slight floral overtones
Odour intensity: low
Evaporation rate/blending classification: top note (see page 143 for a definition of the term 'note')

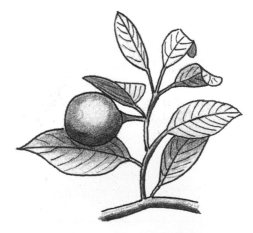

Figure 6.7 Bergamot

Therapeutic Uses

- **Digestive system** – dyspepsia, flatulence, colic, indigestion
- **Immune system** – colds
- **Nervous system** – anxiety, depression and stress–related problems
- **Respiratory system** – asthma, bronchitis, catarrh, coughs
- **Skin care** – acne, oily and congested skins
- **Urinary system** – infections such as cystitis, thrush

Psycho-aromatherapeutic Uses
Uplifting on the mind and spirit
Anger, anxiety, depression, despair, grief, lack of confidence, lack of courage, nervous tension, negativity, worry.

⚠ **Safety data** – Bergamot increases photosensitivity of the skin. Avoid direct contact with sunlight after using this oil.

Black Pepper (*Piper nigrum*)

Plant origin: crushed berries of the vine-like shrub

Method of extraction: steam distillation

Evaporation rate/blending classification: middle note

Aroma characteristics: very sharp, spicy and hot aroma

Odour intensity: high

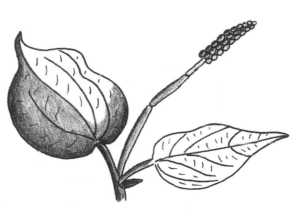

Figure 6.8 Black pepper

Therapeutic Uses

- ■ **Circulation** – poor circulation, anaemia
- ■ **Digestive system** – colic, constipation, diarrhoea, loss of appetite, nausea
- ■ **Immune system** – colds, flu, viral infections
- ■ **Muscular** – muscular aches and pains, poor muscle tone, joint pain and stiffness

Psycho-aromatherapeutic Uses
Fortifying and clearing to the mind
Indifference, lethargy, melancholy, mental fatigue.

⚠ **Safety data** – Black Pepper should be used in low concentrations as it may cause skin irritation.

Chamomile – Roman (*Anthemnis nobilis*)

Plant origin: flowers
Method of extraction: steam distillated
Evaporation rate/blending classification: middle note
Aroma characteristics: a strong apple like aroma, sweet and warm
Odour intensity: very high

Therapeutic Uses

- **Digestive system** – colic, dyspepsia, indigestion, nausea
- **Hormonal** – menstrual and menopausal problems
- **Muscular system** – muscular aches and dull pain
- **Nervous system** – headache, migraine, insomnia, nervous tension and stress related problems
- **Skin care** – allergies, dry and sensitive skins, inflammatory skin conditions
- **Urinary system** – cystitis

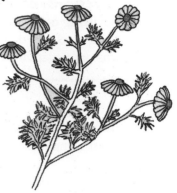

Figure 6.9 Chamomile

Psycho-aromatherapeutic Uses
Calming and soothing on the mind
Anger, anxiety, calming, depression, fear, hysteria, irritability, melancholy, overactive mind, sensitivity, tension, weepiness, excessive worry.

⚠ **Safety data** – it is advisable to avoid using Roman Chamomile in the early stages of pregnancy. Use in low concentrations as it may cause skin irritation.

Clary Sage (*Salvia sclarea*)

Plant origin: herb
Method of extraction: steam distillation
Evaporation rate/blending classification: middle note
Aroma characteristics: a heavy, herbal and nutty aroma
Odour intensity: medium

Therapeutic Uses

- **Circulatory system** – high blood pressure
- **Digestive system** – colic, dyspepsia, constipation, flatulence, intestinal cramps
- **Hormonal system** – pre-menstrual syndrome, menstrual problems (scanty or painful), menopause
- **Muscular system** – muscular aches and pains
- **Nervous system** – migraine, insomnia, debility, stress–related problems
- **Respiratory system** – asthma, bronchitis, throat infections
- **Skin care** – acne and oily skins

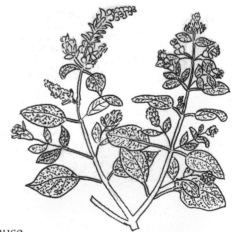

Figure 6.10 Clary sage

Psycho-aromatherapeutic Uses

Balancing to the mood

Anxiety, depression (post-natal, pre-menstrual and menopausal), fear, guilt, moodiness, negativity, obsessional behaviour, panic, paranoia, rage, restlessness, worry.

⚠ **Safety data** – Avoid use of clary sage during pregnancy. Avoid alcohol as it may cause drowsiness in combination with the oil.

Eucalyptus (*Eucalyptus globulus*)

Plant origin: leaves and twigs of the tree
Method of extraction: steam distillation
Evaporation rate/blending classification: top note
Aroma characteristics: clear, sharp, piercing and penetrating aroma; camphoraceous with a woody undertone
Odour intensity: high

Therapeutic Uses

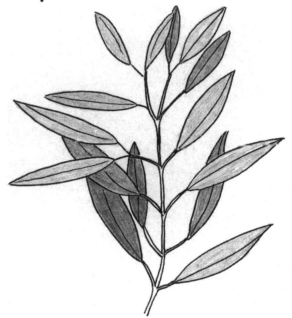

- **Circulatory system** – poor circulation
- **Immune system** – coughs, flu
- **Muscular system** – aches and pains, joint pain
- **Nervous system** : debility, headaches
- **Respiratory system** – asthma, bronchitis, catarrh, coughs, congestion in the head, sinusitis, sore throat
- **Skin care** – healing to the skin
- **Urinary system** – cystitis

Figure 6.11 Eucalyptus

Psycho-aromatherapeutic Uses

Clearing to the head

Addiction, bitterness, guilt, loneliness, moodiness, resentment.

⚠ **Safety data** – Eucalyptus is a powerful oil and should be used in low concentrations. May antidote homeopathic preparations due to its strong odour.

Frankincense (*Boswellia carteri*)

Plant origin: resin of the tree
Method of extraction: steam distillation
Evaporation rate/blending classification:
base note
Aroma characteristics: woody and spicy fragrance
Odour intensity: high

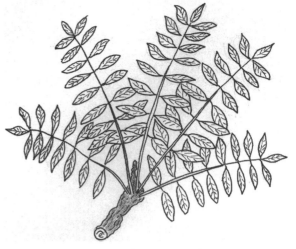

Therapeutic Uses

- **Hormonal** – menstrual problems
- **Immune system** – colds
- **Nervous system** – anxiety, nervous tension, stress-related problems
- **Respiratory system** – asthma, bronchitis, catarrh, coughs, laryngitis
- **Skin care** – regenerating on mature skins, acne, abscesses, scars and blemishes
- **Urinary system** – cystitis

Figure 6.12 Frankincense

Psycho-aromatherapeutic Uses

Helps release emotional blockages

Anger, apprehension, fear, grief, hopelessness, insecurity, irritability, lack of faith, nervous tension, remorse (dwelling on the past), tearfulness, vulnerability, worry.

⚠ **Safety data** – Best avoided in the first trimester of pregnancy.

Geranium (*Pelargonium graveolens*)

Plant origin: leaves of the pelargonium (plant)
Method of extraction: steam distillation
Evaporation rate/blending classification:
middle note
Aroma characteristics: strong sweet and heavy aroma, reminiscent of Rose but with minty overtones
Odour intensity: high

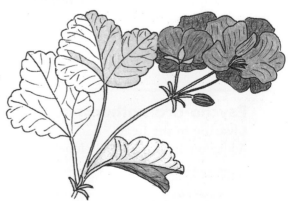

Therapeutic Uses

- **Circulatory system** – poor circulation

Figure 6.13 Geranium

- **Hormonal system** – pre-menstrual syndrome, menopausal problems
- **Lymphatic system** – fluid retention, cellulite
- **Nervous system** – nervous tension and stress-related problems
- **Skin care** – effective on balancing all skin types, especially dry and oily

---

Psycho-aromatherapeutic Uses
Balancing to the mind

Anxiety, confusion, depression (particularly linked to hormones), mental lethargy, moodiness, sadness, tearfulness.

⚠ **Safety data** – May cause irritation to sensitive skins; may cause restlessness if used excessively.

Jasmine (*Jasminum officinale*)

Plant origin: flowers
Method of extraction: solvent extraction
Evaporation rate/blending classification: base note
Aroma characteristics: very sweet, flowery and heavy aroma
Odour intensity: very high

Therapeutic Uses

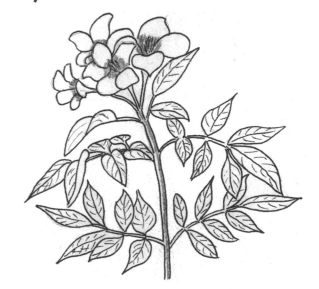

- **Hormonal system** – reproductive problems, menstrual pain, labour pain
- **Muscular system** – muscular aches and pains, stiffness
- **Nervous system** – depression, nervous exhaustion, stress-related problems
- **Respiratory system** – coughs, colds, laryngitis
- **Skin care** – effective on most skin types, especially the hot, dry and sensitive skins

Figure 6.14 Jasmin

Psycho-aromatherapeutic Uses
Confidence booster

Confusion, fear, depression, inhibition, lack of confidence, lack of self-worth, lack of interest, lack of trust, nervous tension, sadness.

⚠ **Safety data** – No known hazards if used in sensible proportions.

Juniper (*Juniperus communis*)

Plant origin: berries of the tree
Method of extraction: distillation
Evaporation rate/blending classification: middle note
Aroma characteristics: clear, refreshing, slightly woody aroma
Odour intensity: medium

Therapeutic Uses

- **Circulatory system** – poor circulation
- **Hormonal system** – menstrual problems
- **Lymphatic system** – fluid retention, tissue toxication
- **Muscular system** – muscular aches and pains, stiffness
- **Nervous system** – anxiety and nervous tension, stress-related problems
- **Skin care** – effective for acne, congested and oily skins

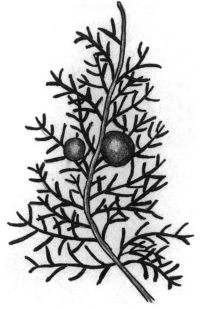

Figure 6.15 Juniper

Psycho-aromatherapeutic Uses
Cleansing to the mind and spirit
Addiction, confusion, feelings of worthlessness, feelings of being emotionally drained, guilt, fear, obsession, restlessness, withdrawal.

⚠ **Safety data** – Best avoided during pregnancy. Use in moderation as it can be very stimulating.

Lavender (*Lavendula officinalis, Lavendula augustifolia*)

Plant origin: flowers
Method of extraction: steam distillation
Evaporation rate/blending classification: middle
Aroma characteristics: powerful herbal/floral aroma
Odour intensity: medium

Therapeutic Uses

- **Circulatory system** – high blood pressure, heart conditions
- **Digestive system** – colic, dyspepsia, flatulence, nausea
- **Hormonal system** – pre-menstrual syndrome
- **Immune system** – colds, flu

- **Muscular system** – muscular aches and pains, joint pain
- **Nervous system** – depression, headache, insomnia, migraine, nervous tension and stress-related problems
- **Respiratory system** – asthma, bronchitis, coughs, sinusitis
- **Skin care** – all skin types, very healing and regenerating on all skins

---

Psycho-aromatherapeutic Uses
Calming and soothing to the mind
Anger, anxiety, despondency, depression, emotional instability, fear, hysteria, impatience, irritation, mood swings, negative thoughts, panic, paranoia, worry.

 Safety data – Best avoided during the early stages of pregnancy.

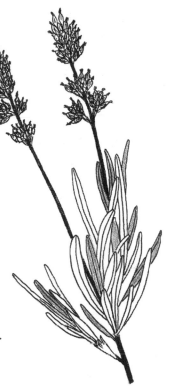

Figure 6.16 Lavender

Lemon (*Citrus limonum*)

Plant origin: rind of fruit
Method of extraction: expression
Evaporation rate/blending classification: top note
Aroma characteristics: refreshing, sharp, citrus aroma
Odour intensity: high

Therapeutic Uses

- **Circulation system** – poor circulation
- **Digestive system** – dyspepsia, bloatedness
- **Immune system** – colds, flu and infections
- **Respiratory system** – asthma, bronchitis, catarrh, sore throat
- **Skin care** – especially effective for oily skins

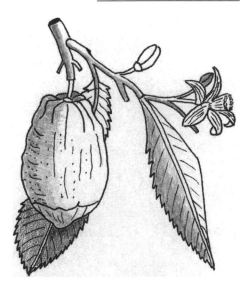

Figure 6.17 Lemon

Psycho-aromatherapeutic Uses
Uplifting on the spirit
Mental fatigue, depression, fear.

⚠ **Safety data** – may cause skin irritation and sensitisation in some individuals. The expressed essential oil is phototoxic; do not use on skin exposed to direct sunlight.

Marjoram (*Origanum marjorana*)

Plant origin: herb
Method of extraction: distillation
Evaporation rate/blending classification: middle note
Aroma characteristics: deeply penetrating, peppery, nutty, spicy and warming aroma
Odour intensity: medium

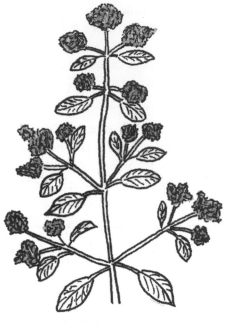

Therapeutic Uses

- **Circulatory system** – high blood pressure, heart conditions
- **Digestive system** – colic, constipation, dyspepsia, flatulence
- **Hormonal system** – menstrual problems, premenstrual syndrome
- **Immune system** – colds
- **Muscular system** – muscular aches and stiffness, joint pain
- **Nervous system** – headaches, migraine, insomnia, nervous tension and stress related problems

Figure 6.18 Marjoram

- **Respiratory system** – asthma, bronchitis, coughs

Psycho-aromatherapeutic Uses
Soothing and fortifying to the mind
Anxiety, depression, fear, grief, loneliness, nervous tension.

⚠ **Safety data** – best avoided during pregnancy.

Neroli (*Citrus aurantium*)

Plant origin: orange blossom flowers
Method of extraction: distillation
Evaporation rate/blending classification: middle to base note
Aroma characteristics: very sweet, floral aroma with a bitter undertone
Odour intensity: medium

Therapeutic Uses

- **Circulatory system** – poor circulation

- **Digestive system** – colic, flatulence (stress related digestive problems such as irritable bowel syndrome)
- **Hormonal system** – premenstrual syndrome
- **Nervous system** – anxiety, depression, nervous tension
- **Skin care** – effective for all skin types especially the dry, sensitive and mature skins

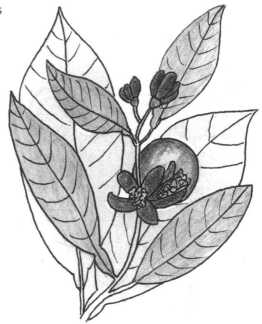

Figure 6.19 Neroli

Psycho-aromatherapeutic Uses
Reliever of extreme stress
Anxiety, apprehension, desperation, emotional trauma, fear, nervous tension.

 Safety data – no known hazards.

Orange – Sweet (*Citrus Aurantium var dulcis/var. sinensis*)

Plant origin: rind of fruit
Method of extraction: expressed
Evaporation rate/blending classification: top to middle note
Aroma characteristics: sweet fruity aroma, zesty and warm
Odour intensity: medium

Therapeutic Uses

- **Digestive system** – indigestion, constipation, stress related disorders such as irritable bowel syndrome)

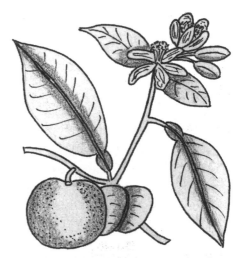

Figure 6.20 Orange – Sweet

- **Immune system** – colds and flu
- **Lymphatic system** – fluid retention
- **Nervous system** – nervous tension and stress related problems
- **Skin care** – effective for dull, congested and oily skins

---

Psycho-aromatherapeutic Uses
Comforting and warming to the spirit
Anxiety, depression, emotional exhaustion.

⚠ **Safety data** – no known hazards.

Peppermint (*Mentha piperita*)

Plant origin: herb
Method of extraction: distillation
Evaporation rate/blending classification: top note
Aroma characteristics: strong, sharp piercing menthol aroma
Odour intensity: very high

Therapeutic Uses

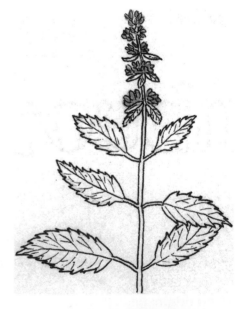

- **Digestive system** – colic, cramp, dyspepsia, flatulence and nausea
- **Immune system** – colds and flu
- **Muscular system** – muscular pain, joint pain
- **Nervous system** – headaches, migraine, nervous stress
- **Respiratory system** – asthma, bronchitis, sinusitis
- **Skin care** – congested skins

Figure 6.21 Peppermint

Psycho-aromatherapeutic Uses
Reviving to the spirit
Depression, mental fatigue.

⚠ **Safety data** – use in moderation as it is a very stimulating oil. May cause sensitisation due to menthol constituent. Best avoided if homeopathic remedies being taken.

Rose (*Rosa damascena/centifolia*)

Plant origin: petals of flowers
Method of extraction: solvent extraction/distillation
Evaporation rate/blending classification: base note
Aroma characteristics: rose otto has a sweet and mellow aroma with a hint of vanilla, rose absolute has a deep, rich and sweet honey-rose aroma
Odour intensity: very high

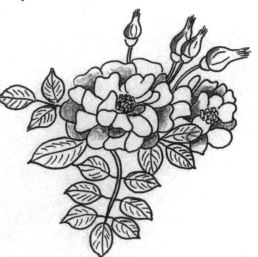

Therapeutic Uses

- **Circulatory system** – poor circulation
- **Hormonal system** – menstrual problems, premenstrual syndrome, menopause
- **Nervous system** – depression, insomnia, nervous tension, stress related problems
- **Respiratory system** – asthma, coughs, hay fever

Figure 6.22 Rose

- **Skin care** – all skin types especially dry, ageing and sensitive skins

Psycho-aromatherapeutic Uses
Confidence booster
Bereavement and grief, emotional trauma, insecurity, lack of confidence, lack of self worth, melancholia, nervous tension.

 Safety data – no known hazards.

Rosemary (*Rosmarinus officinalis*)

Plant origin: herb
Method of extraction: distillation
Evaporation rate/blending classification: middle note
Aroma characteristics: strong, herbal aroma with a clear, warm and penetrating note
Odour intensity: high

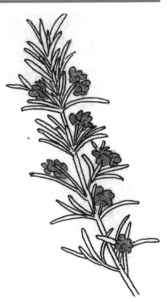

Therapeutic Uses

- **Circulatory system** – poor circulation
- **Immune system** – colds, flu
- **Lymphatic system** – fluid retention
- **Muscular system** – muscular aches and pains, joint pain

Figure 6.23 Rosemary

- **Nervous system** – debility, headaches, mental fatigue, nervous exhaustion
- **Respiratory system** – asthma, bronchitis, sinusitis
- **Skin care** – especially effective for oily skin and scalp disorders

---

Psycho-aromatherapeutic Uses
Uplifting and energising to the mind

Anguish, anxiety, confusion, depression, doubt, emotional numbness, nervous debility.

⚠ **Safety data** – best avoided during pregnancy. Due to its highly stimulating actions it is best avoided for epilepsy sufferer and those with high blood pressure.

Sandalwood (*Santalum album*)

Plant origin: heartwood of the tree
Method of extraction: distillation
Evaporation rate/blending classification:
base note
Aroma characteristics: very subtle, woody and
exotic aroma
Odour intensity: medium

Therapeutic Uses

- **Digestive system** – diarrhoea, nausea
- **Immune system** – colds, flu, infections
- **Lymphatic system** – cellulite
- **Nervous system** – anxiety, depression, insomnia, nervous tension, stress related problems
- **Respiratory system** – bronchitis, catarrh, cough, laryngitis, sore throats
- **Skin care** – effective for dry, dehydrated, oily skins and acne
- **Urinary system** – cystitis

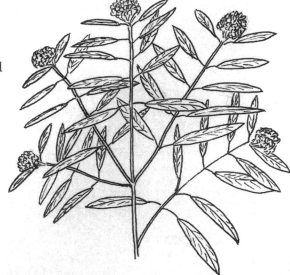

Figure 6.24 Sandalwood

Psycho-aromatherapeutic Uses
Fortifies the spirit

Apprehension, emotional exhaustion, insecurity, fear, lack of courage, nervous tension, sensitivity, shyness, tearfulness, timidity, weakness of spirit.

⚠ **Safety data** – no known hazards.

Teatree (*Malaleuca alternifolia*)

Plant origin: leaves of the tree
Method of extraction: distillation
Evaporation rate/blending classification: top note
Aroma characteristics: strong antiseptic aroma
Odour intensity: very high

Therapeutic Uses

- **Immune system** – colds, flu, infections
- **Respiratory system** – asthma, bronchitis, catarrh, coughs, sinusitis
- **Skin care** – oily skins
- **Urinary system** – cystitis, thrush

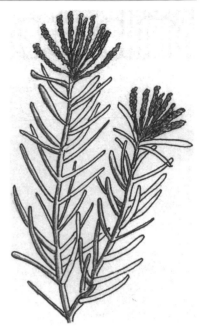

> **Psycho-aromatherapeutic Uses**
> **Psychic protector**
> Fear, hypochondria, hysteria, negativity, shock.

Figure 6.25 Teatree

⚠ **Safety data** – may cause irritation and sensitisation to some skins.

Ylang Ylang (*Cananga odorata*)

Plant origin: flowers
Method of extraction: distillation
Evaporation rate/blending classification: base note
Aroma characteristics: very sweet heavy, floral and exotic aroma
Odour intensity: high

Therapeutic Uses

- **Circulatory system** – high blood pressure
- **Hormonal system** – hormonal problems
- **Nervous system** – anxiety, depression, insomnia, nervous tension, stress related problems
- **Skin care** – oily and dry skins

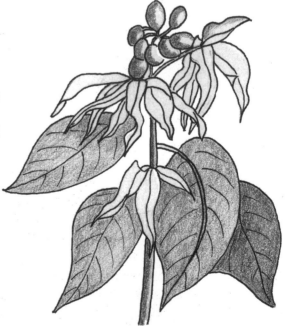

Figure 6.26 Ylang ylang

Psycho-aromatherapeutic Uses
Confidence booster
Anger, insecurity, fear, frustration, panic, introversion, lack of confidence, jealousy, sensitivity, stubbornness.

⚠ **Safety data** – may cause sensitisation in some skins. Use in low concentrations as its heady aroma may cause headaches and nausea.

AROMATHERAPY AND SKIN CARE

The use of essential oils in skin care is remarkable. These oils enhance the protective functions of the skin because the majority of them are antiseptic. Essential oils have the ability to penetrate the skin due to their small molecular size and can be absorbed into the skin to encourage healing and cell regeneration. Since some essential oils have molecular structures that are similar to hormones, they can act on our endocrine system, which in turn regulates the functions of the skin.

Essential Oils for Different Skin Types

SKIN TYPE	RECOMMENDED OILS
Dry	Roman Chamomile, Geranium, Jasmin, Lavender, Neroli, Rose, Sandalwood, Ylang Ylang
Oily	Bergamot, Clary Sage, Geranium, Juniper, Lavender, Lemon, Rosemary, Sweet Orange, Teatree, Sandalwood, Ylang Ylang
Mature	Frankincense, Geranium, Lavender, Neroli, Rose
Sensitive	Roman Chamomile, Jasmin, Lavender, Neroli, Rose, Sandalwood

BLENDING

When essential oils are blended together, they act in synergy so that the combination becomes more than the sum of the individual parts. The art of aromatherapy lies in creating a synergistic blend that suits the individual needs of a client. Blending is an art which takes practice. The key to successful blending is to have a good working knowledge of the effects, characteristics and therapeutic properties of the oils, as well as having personal experience of using them. As there is such a diversity in the range of essential oils, there are endless blending combinations.

Factors to Consider When Blending
Proportions
A safe and effective ratio of essential oil to carrier oil is usually 2%. For instance, if preparing 20 ml of carrier oil you could add up to 10 drops (approx 0.4 ml) of essential oil to the carrier. In some instances it may be necessary to blend a lower percentage dilution, such as for pregnant women, clients with sensitive skins or for babies and children.

Notes
The classification of essential oils by 'notes' originates from the perfumery industry. It is useful to take account of this system of classification in order to create a well balanced blend.

- A **top note** is highly volatile and, generally, will give the first impression of smell in a blend. Top notes are usually fast-acting.
- A **middle note** is less volatile and will help to balance a blend.
- A **base note** is the least volatile and will act as a fixative in the blend so that aroma will last longer.

Compatibility
Certain essential oils are mutually enhancing and blend well together, whereas others may have an inhibiting effect on each other. There are no golden rules for blending compatible oils; personal experimentation is the only way of finding which oils blend successfully. It is important to remember that the proportion of each oil has a bearing on how the blend smells.

Odour Intensity
This is an important factor to consider. Some oils are highly odorous and may predominate. These should be used in small proportions in order to create a balanced blend.

Client Preference
As smell is largely subjective, it is important to take account of the client's preference. If in doubt as to which oils to use, ask the client what types of aroma they prefer (i.e. floral, citrus etc.).

Cost Effectiveness
It is important to avoid wastage by only blending as much as is needed for an individual treatment. An aromatherapy massage treatment is not necessarily improved by blending several oils for the sake of it, when fewer oils may suit the purpose equally well. If the therapist uses a maximum of three or four essential oils in a blend, the client will be able to appreciate each individual aroma, whilst still benefiting from a synergistic blend. Depending on the size of the client and their skin type, it is usual to need between 20–30 ml of carrier oil for a full aromatherapy massage and between 10–15 mls for an aromatherapy massage to specific body parts.

Client Type
For clients with special needs, such as pregnant women, children or those with sensitive skin, it is recommended that a lower dilution of 1% is used. A careful choice of oils would also be necessary (see page 119 for guidance).

Client Need

Client needs will always be the primary factor when making the final selection of oils. It is important to assess the main, presenting problems, along with the client's emotional state, so that the client's needs and objectives for the treatment are met.

Client Skin Type

If the client has a sensitive skin or is prone to allergies, it may influence the oils selected, in order to avoid any adverse reactions.

Area to be treated

Unless the client is prone to sensitivity and allergies, it is usual practice to use a 2% dilution of essential oils in carrier oil for therapeutic bodywork. However, when working on more sensitive areas such as the face it is recommended that a lower dilution of 1% is used.

CARRIER OILS

Carrier oils are not just blending agents for essential oils, they also have their own valuable therapeutic properties. Where it is possible, it is important to buy **cold pressed** carrier oils as these retain their natural constituents. However, some oils are partially refined in order to avoid difficulties when using or storing. Grapeseed oil, for instance, in its natural state is very dark in colour with a strong odour. The choice of carrier will be largely dependent on the client's skin type.

> ***KEY NOTE*** Always check the sensitivity of the client's skin and ask whether they have any allergies (to nut or wheat for instance) before using a carrier oil.

Alphabetical List of Carrier Oils

Nut-based and wheat-based oils are identified with an asterisk (*).

Apricot Kernel

Source: extracted from the seed kernel of the fruit.
Therapeutic properties: this oil is high in Vitamin A and B and, therefore, aids healing and rejuvenation of skin cells. It has a light, fine texture and is easily absorbed. A popular choice for facial massage.
Uses: suitable for all skin types, especially dry, sensitive, inflamed and prematurely ageing skin.

Avocado

Source: the large seed and flesh of the fruit.
Therapeutic properties: soothing, relieves itching. Contains protein, lecithin, essential fatty acids, vitamins A, B and D. This oil is highly penetrative.
Uses: suitable for all skin types, especially dry, dehydrated, undernourished, ageing or sensitive skins. Has a rich, heavy quality and should be added in small proportions (10%) to a lighter carrier.

Calendula
Source: from macerated flowers.
Therapeutic properties: anti-inflammatory, softening, soothing, moisturising and healing.
Uses: suitable for all skin types, especially dry and sensitive skins.

Carrot
Source: orange carrot root macerated in a vegetable oil.
Therapeutic properties: rich in beta-carotene, anti-inflammatory, rejuvenating, anti-ageing.
Uses: suitable for ageing skins and scar tissue. Use in very small quantities and dilute well with another carrier.

Grapeseed
Source: the grape pips of the fruit.
Therapeutic properties: gentle emollient, contains linoleic acid, protein and a small proportion of vitamin E; is free from cholesterol.
Uses: suitable for all skin types. Is light and penetrates the skin quickly.

*Jojoba
Source: from the bean-like nuts
Therapeutic properties: anti-inflammatory and highly penetrative. The chemical structure resembles sebum and contains a waxy substance that mimics collagen. Rich in vitamin E, protein and minerals. Is a natural moisturiser.
Uses: suitable for all skin types including oily, combination, acne skins and inflamed skin. This oil has a light and fine texture and is suitable for both facial and body massage.

Rose Hip
Source: the seeds of the fruit
Therapeutic properties: high in vitamin C, very regenerating and healing. Very useful in scar tissue repair and for healing of burns.
Uses: suitable for mature and ageing skins, stretch marks, scarred skin and burns. Dilute with another carrier (50%).

St John's Wort
Source: macerated flowers and leaves
Therapeutic properties: anti-inflammatory, astringent, soothing and healing.
Uses: suitable for all skin types especially dry and sensitive. Is an excellent carrier for oils used to treat aching muscles and inflammation, also nerve-related pain.

*Sweet Almond
Source: from the nut of the *Prunus amygdalus* (sweet almond tree).
Therapeutic properties: soothing and calming, helps relieve itching. Contains vitamins A, B1, B2, B6, E and is rich in protein. Contains a high proportion of unsaturated fatty acids.
Uses: suitable for all skin types, especially dry, ageing and inflamed skins.

*Wheatgerm
Source: from the golden germ of the wheat grain.
Therapeutic properties: is high in vitamins A, D and E and is a natural anti-oxidant. Is soothing, nourishing and healing. Helps skin cells regenerate and skin keep soft and supple. Healing of scars, burns and stretch marks.

Uses: suitable for all skin types, especially ageing and inflamed skins. Use in small quantities as an addition to another carrier.

How to Blend Oils for Aromatherapy Massage

The equipment needed in order to blend essential oils includes:

- a clear glass or plastic measuring cup (marked in mls)
- selected essential oils to suit the client's needs
- selected carrier oils to suit the client's needs and skin type
- selection of dark glass bottles, i.e. 5 mls, 10 mls, 15 mls and 25 mls
- glass rod for stirring
- labels.

Method

1. The amount of carrier oil or oils required for the massage are measured into a blending cup, or they are measured directly into the dark glass bottle up to the shoulder level.
2. A number of selected essential oils are then added one at a time, drop by drop, in the correct ratio.
3. If blending in a cup, it is necessary to stir the blend with a glass rod or other suitable implement such as a spatula.
4. If blending in a bottle. The lid should be placed on the bottle and then it can be shaken to disperse the essential oils into the carrier. The bottle should be labelled.

> **KEY NOTE** Care should be taken when blending essential oils that the correct tops are placed onto the correct bottles. It is advisable to place a small label on the top of the bottles for easy identification when replacing tops.

CONSULTATION FOR AROMATHERAPY MASSAGE

A consultation for aromatherapy massage will cover the following areas:

- the client's medical history and any current medical treatment
- their main presenting problems and physical and emotional state
- general health, including generally immunity, energy levels, stress levels, sleep patterns
- lifestyle patterns, including diet and fluid intake, smoking habits, alcohol consumption, stress levels, family situation, work situation, exercise levels, hobbies and methods of relaxation
- client declaration and signature.

> **KEY NOTE** The aromatherapy consultation from is slightly different to the massage consultation form. It is designed to illicit a specific aromatherapy treatment plan.

An example of an aromatherapy consultation form

AROMATHERAPY CONSULTATION FORM

Client Note

The following information is required for your safety and to benefit your health. Whilst essential oils and massage are totally safe when administered professionally by a trained aromatherapist, there are certain contra-indications which may require special attention.

The following details will be treated in the strictest of confidence. If may, however, be necessary for you to consult your GP before any aromatherapy treatment can be given.

Date of initial consultation: _____   Client ref. No. _____

Personal Details

Name: _____   Title: Mr/Mrs/Miss/Ms/Other

Address: _____

_____

Telephone Number Daytime: _____   Evening: _____

Date of Birth: _____   Occupation: _____

Medical details

Name of Doctor: _____   Surgery: _____

Address: _____

_____

Telephone Number: _____

Do you have/have you ever suffered with any of the following conditions?
(Please give dates and details)

Skin Complaints

			Dates and Details
Acne	Y	N	_____
Allergies	Y	N	_____
Dermatitis	Y	N	_____
Eczema	Y	N	_____
Psoriasis	Y	N	_____
Scabies	Y	N	_____
Other	Y	N	_____

Circulatory Disorders

Dates and Details

Heart condition	Y	N	_____
High or low blood pressure	Y	N	_____
Oedema	Y	N	_____
Thrombosis or embolism	Y	N	_____
Varicose veins	Y	N	_____

Digestive Problems

Dates and Details

Constipation	Y	N	_____
Indigestion	Y	N	_____
Colitis	Y	N	_____
Candida	Y	N	_____
Irritable bowel syndrome	Y	N	_____
Other	Y	N	_____

Urinary Problems

Dates and Details

Cystitis	Y	N	_____
Thrush	y	N	_____
Other	Y	N	_____

Nervous or Stress-related Problems

Dates and Details

Any nervous dysfunction	Y	N	_____
Epilepsy	Y	N	_____
Anxiety	Y	N	_____
Depression	Y	N	_____
Headaches	Y	N	_____
Migraine	Y	N	_____
Insomnia	Y	N	_____
Nervous tension	Y	N	_____
Other	Y	N	_____

Endocrine Disorders

Dates and Details

Diabetes	Y	N	_____
Thyroid Problems?	Y	N	_____

Other Health Related Information

Dates and Details

Have you had a recent operation?   Y   N   _____

Have you had a potentially fatal or terminal   Y   N   _____
condition?

Female Clients

Dates and Details

Is it possible that you may be pregnant?   Y   N   _____

Any complications with the pregnancy?   Y   N   _____

Do you have pre-menstrual tension?   Y   N   _____

Menopausal problems?   Y   N   _____

Problems with periods?   Y   N   _____

Other?   Y   N   _____

Current medical treatment: _____

_____

_____

Current medication (list dosages): _____

_____

Section for use by therapist

GP referral required: Yes ( )   No ( )

Clearance form sent: Yes ( )   No ( )   Date:_____

Clearance form received: Yes ( )   No ( )   Date:_____

General State of Health and Lifestyle

Do you smoke?   Yes ( ) average per day _____   No ( )

Do you drink alcohol?   Yes ( ) average daily consumption _____   No ( )

How many glasses of water do you drink daily? _____

How would you describe your diet? _____

General immunity: Good ( )   Average ( )   Poor ( )

Energy levels: High ( )   Average ( )   Low ( )

Stress levels: High ( )   Medium ( )   Low ( )

Sleep pattern: Good ( )   Average ( )   Poor ( )

Exercise undertaken/lifestyle:_____

_____

Do you follow a regular exercise programme?   Yes ( )   No ( )

_____

Details_____

_____

Do you have any hobbies/time set aside for relaxation?   Yes ( )   No ( )

Details_____

_____

Have you ever had an aromatherapy treatment before?   Yes ( )   No ( )

If yes, please give brief details of previous treatments and success: _____

_____

Are you currently having any other forms of alternative or complementary therapy treatment? (please state) _____

_____

Client declaration

I declare that the information that I have given, is true and correct and that, as far as I am aware, I can undertake treatment with this establishment without any adverse effects. I have been fully informed about contra-indications and am willing, therefore, to proceed. I understand that aromatherapy is not a substitute for medical advice and/or treatment.

Client's signature: _____   Date: _____

Therapist's signature: _____   Date: _____

AROMATHERAPY TREATMENT RECORD

An aromatherapy treatment record will include the following:

- the date of treatment
- feedback from the last treatment if applicable, noting client response and any changes or improvements in the client's condition
- any new information relating to the client's condition and which is required to update the original consultation form
- treatment objectives for the session and any specific client needs
- an outline of the proposed treatment, taking account of length of treatment, areas for treatment and cost
- the carrier oil and essential oils chosen, stating quantity used and reasons for choice

- a manual and visual evaluation of the client's tissues, noting any areas of tension, erythema, areas of fluid retention, blockages in the nerve pathways etc.
- known contra-actions, effects and advice given
- after care advice given
- home care advice given, along with products to use
- outcome and evaluation of the treatment
- recommendations for future treatment.

KEY NOTE It is very important to review the client's treatment plan for aromatherapy massage at regular intervals. Care should be taken not to use the same blend of oils for an extended period of time, to avoid building up sensitivity.

AROMATHERAPY MASSAGE TECHNIQUES

Aromatherapy massage combines the use of the Swedish massage techniques of effleurage, petrissage, friction and vibration, but omits the more vigorous movements, such as tapotement (see pages 99–101). In addition aromatherapy is usually performed more slowly than therapeutic massage and it includes specialised techniques such as attention to pressure points.

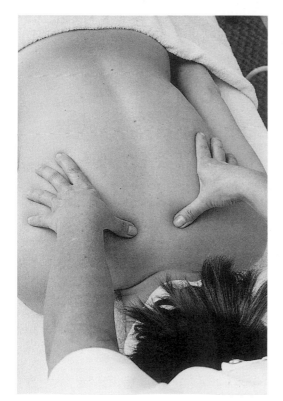

Figure 6.27 Pressures on the back

Pressures

These techniques are performed by applying pressure along the nerve tracts or meridians with the thumbs and fingers. Pressure is applied as the client breathes out.

These specialised pressures techniques are a form of 'energy' massage and are designed to:
- increase the blood supply to the tissues and promote cell renewal
- stimulate the nerves and help clear energy blocks
- ease congestion of the nervous system by relieving tension from the nerve tracts.

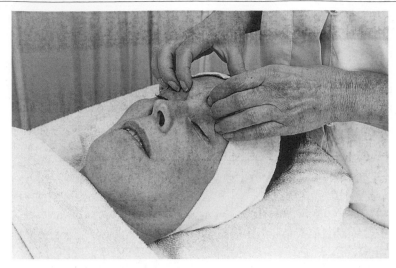

Figure 6.28 Pressures on the face

AROMATHERAPY MASSAGE PROCEDURE

A full aromatherapy massage treatment will typically include massage to the body, the face and scalp. It may take between one hour and one and a half hours depending on the needs of the client. For practical reasons, a client may be unable to have a full treatment and may require localised massage to specific areas.

Whatever form of massage treatment is given, it is essential that it is adapted to suit the individual needs of the client at the time. As client needs will vary from one treatment to the next, it is important to review the treatment plans on each occasion.

REACTIONS TO AROMATHERAPY MASSAGE

The reactions to an aromatherapy massage may be similar to the reactions to a therapeutic massage. The main difference will come from the effects of the oils used. Clients often feel very tired and deeply relaxed after an aromatherapy massage, as the body is encouraged to relax and heal. Some clients may feel emotionally uplifted and revitalised as blockages in the energy pathways have been cleared.

It is important for an aromatherapist to monitor carefully a client's reaction to the aromatherapy massage and the effects of the oils used in order to evaluate the effectiveness of the treatment. The effect of the treatment and the oils may be cumulative and must be assessed over a period of time.

Contra-actions to Aromatherapy Massage

■ **Skin reaction** – this may occur if the client's skin is sensitive to an essential oil or carrier oil. If a skin reaction occurs, the affected areas should be washed with warm water in order to remove as much of the product as possible. If the condition continues, the client should seek medical advice. It is important to always record any skin reaction in order to avoid exposure to the substance on subsequent occasions.

■ **Feeling faint or dizzy** – this may occur due to the deep, relaxing effects of the massage and the effects of the oils. Clients should be advised to get up gradually to avoid feeling faint and dizzy.

■ **Sickness or nausea** – some clients may experience a feeling of nausea or sickness during or after the treatment. If this occurs during the treatment, it may be advisable to stop the massage to avoid exacerbating the effects.

> **KEY NOTE** It is important for an aromatherapist to record on the client's treatment records all contra-actions as they occur, or as they are reported.

AFTER CARE ADVICE

The following advice should be given to a client following aromatherapy massage:

■ avoid washing the skin or bathing for at least 8 hours following treatment (absorption may take as little as 15 minutes and as long as 12 hours)

■ avoid direct exposure to strong sunlight (artificial and natural) for at least 8 hours following treatment with phototoxic oils

■ avoid alcohol and smoking in order to allow the body to detoxify naturally

■ drink plenty of water to assist the natural detoxification process

■ eat a light diet in order to encourage healing and detoxification

■ enjoy rest and relaxation in order to maximise the effects of the treatment and avoid overexerting the body.

In addition to the above advice, an aromatherapist may wish to advise on the following for long-term benefits:

■ lifestyle patterns

■ the importance of regular treatment

■ how the effects of the treatment may be maintained at home

It is important that clients are advised correctly about the use of essential oils at home. It can be damaging for clients to use oils at home without professional advice. This is because:

■ excessive exposure can have adverse effects

■ clients may not appreciate or recognise the effects

■ using essential oils for a purpose other than that which has been agreed can be detrimental to future treatments.

CHAPTER 7

Reflexology

INTRODUCTION

Reflexology is another form of natural healing that is both a science and an art. The science lies in the principle that there are reflex areas in the feet and the hands, which correspond to all parts of the body. The art is in the unique technique applied to the reflex areas by the thumbs and the fingers.

Reflexology is a holistic therapy in that it uses the feet to treat the whole body. It aims to restore balance by increasing the circulation to the internal organs, glands and other parts of the body through the feet. By working on the reflexes of the feet, reflexologists can help to facilitate **homeostasis** (balance in the body fluids) by unblocking energy that stagnates in the feet.

Reflexology is often favoured over other forms of holistic therapy because undressing is not required, other than the removal of socks and shoes, and it can be practised virtually anywhere that is comfortable for the practitioner and the client. Reflexology is becoming well established as a popular complementary therapy. It is an extremely relaxing and non-invasive way of helping to harmonise the body's functions. It helps the body to heal itself by breaking down tension, relieving stress, and improving the blood and nerve supply.

BRIEF HISTORY

Reflexology is thought to have originated over 5000 years ago when pressure therapies, similar to acupuncture, were practised by the Chinese as a preventive medicine. The earliest recording of what is thought to be the origins of reflexology is an Egyptian tomb drawing dated 2330 BC, which illustrates a person applying massage to the soles of the feet of another person. However, it is not really possible to establish the exact relationship between the ancient art that was practised by the Egyptians and modern reflexology.

We do know that reflexology is based on the same principle as acupuncture, but without the use of needles. The link between the ancient art of foot massage and the modern techniques we use today, is the long established principle that there are energy zones running throughout the body, and reflex areas in the feet mirror the organs, glands and corresponding parts of the body. In order to understand reflexology as it is known today, it is important to understand **zone theory** which was the precursor of modern reflexology.

Zone Theory

In the early part of the nineteenth century, Dr William H. Fitzgerald, an American ear nose and throat specialist, began researching into a method of healing which he called 'zone analgesia'. He discovered that when pressure was applied to certain parts of the body, it created an anaesthetic effect. He made use of the clothes pegs, elastic bands and aluminium combs in order to apply pressure to parts of the body in order to achieve pain relief. This lead Dr Fitzgerald to formulate the first chart of the longitudinal zones of the body: he described how the body could be divided into ten longitudinal zones, five on either side of the central line of the body. Dr Fitzgerald's findings were that energy links the organs in each particular zone and, if one area is out of balance, then the whole zone may be affected. He also discovered that the application of pressure to the zones not only helped to relieve pain but also helped to relieve the underlying cause. The pain would often manifest itself at a distance from its origin, having been referred to another part of a zone.

Dr Shelby Riley worked closely with Dr Fitzgerald and developed the zone theory further. Dr Riley is thought to have added horizontal zones across the hands and feet, together with the longitudinal zones in order to determine individual reflexes according to the zone theory.

Eunice Ingham, a physical therapist, worked closely with Dr Riley and used the zone theory in her treatment of many patients. In the early 1930s she began to develop a foot reflex theory. Her extensive experience led her to conclude that the feet were the most responsive areas, as they were extremely sensitive. She determined that the reflexes of the feet were an exact mirror of the organs and parts of the body. She subsequently mapped the entire body on the feet. She also discovered that an alternating pressure on the reflex points gave improved therapeutic effects.

Eunice Ingham documented her findings and the many cases she had treated in her first book *Stories the Feet Can Tell* which was published in 1938. She continued to work tirelessly to promote the benefits of her techniques and travelled extensively to spread the word of reflexology. Eunice Ingham's indisputable contributions to modern reflexology are that she mapped the reflex areas onto the foot according to the anatomical model of the body, she discovered that an alternating pressure was more effective and she helped to promote reflexology as a complementary therapy that was of benefit to the whole community.

Reflexology was introduced to Great Britain in the early 1960s by Doreen Bayly (a student of Eunice Ingham). Doreen Bayly instructed many of the early practitioners in the practice of reflexology. Eunice Ingham's legacy also continues overseas under the direction of her nephew, Dwight Byers, who runs the International Institute of Reflexology in St Petersburg, Florida.

Modern reflexology as it is known today, was born from the initial practice of zone theory and developed to concentrate on the reflex areas of the feet. Reflexology is rooted in the theory that energy pathways begin in the feet and that blockages may lead to ill health and disease.

HOW REFLEXOLOGY WORKS

It is unclear exactly how reflexology works. However, the foundation for the theory is that the body is divided into ten longitudinal zones or nerve pathways, and that these zones run the entire length of the body.

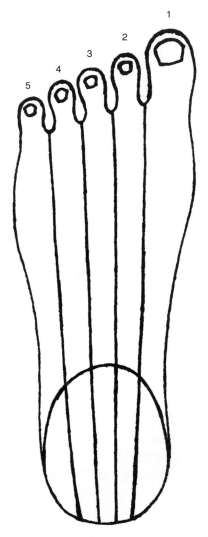

Figure 7.1 The longitudinal zones

> **KEY NOTE** Each zone may be considered as a channel of energy, or 'chi' as described in oriental medicine. Working a zone in the foot with pressure from the thumbs and fingers, can help to release vital energy that may be blocked in any part of the zone and corresponding part of the body.

Reflexology is, therefore, a holistic therapy – it can help to balance the zones and can improve the function of related organs, glands and parts of the body. It is thought that, when the reflexes on the feet are stimulated, an involuntary response is effected in the organs, glands and parts of the body connected by energy pathways to the reflexes. This triggers a reaction in the body to facilitate healing and balance.

The actual physical mechanism of reflexology remains largely unknown, but it is generally accepted that the therapy can have effects on the blood and lymphatic circulation and the nervous system, revitalising and destressing the body so that the natural healing mechanism may be initiated.

BENEFITS AND EFFECTS OF REFLEXOLOGY

- **Improves circulation** – reflexology stimulates the circulation, facilitating better transport of nutrients around the body and encouraging the elimination of waste.
- **Stress reduction** – reflexology can be a powerful antidote to stress. It has been estimated that over 75% of illness is stress-related. Reflexology can help to reduce nerve tension by generating deep relaxation, allowing the body to rest and repair itself.
- **Relaxation** – reflexology provides deep relaxation; relaxation is the first step towards restoring balance in the body.
- **Pain relief** – reflexology can have a positive effect on the nervous system by promoting the release of endorphins, the body's own natural pain-relieving agents. Endorphins are also known to help to elevate the mood.
- **Facilitates homeostasis** – being a holistic therapy, reflexology aims to facilitate better health and well-being by treating the whole body and the whole person through the feet (or hands). Reflexology can help to return the body to state of balance and harmony by encouraging the mind and body to better health.
- **Revitalisation of energy** – by relaxing and opening up the energy pathways in the zones, reflexology can help to clear blockages and revitalise the body with renewed energy.
- **Strengthens the immune system** – reflexology works to initiate the body's own healing forces which often become suppressed through illness, stress and medication. Reflexology helps to improve the body's defences and encourages better immunity.

ANATOMY OF THE FOOT

In order to be able to locate each reflex area accurately on the foot, it is important for a reflexologist to have a good knowledge of the anatomical structure of the foot. The foot provides support for the weight of the body during walking, running and standing.

Each foot contains 26 bones: 7 tarsals, 5 metatarsals and 14 phalanges.

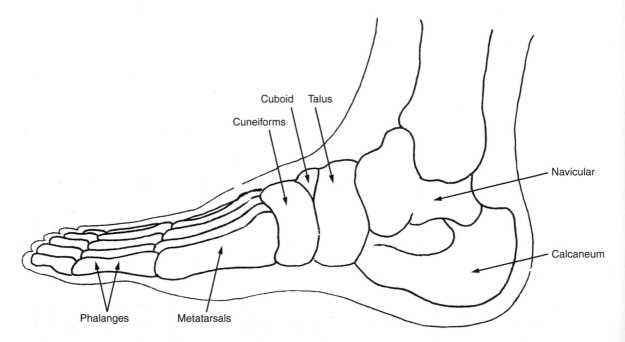

Figure 7.2 The bones of the feet

Tarsals

Each tarsal is an irregular bone that slides minutely over the next bone. Collectively the tarsals form joints and provide motion.

- ■ **Talus** – this is the main tarsal and it bears the weight of the body when standing or walking. It articulates with the tibia and fibula to form the ankle joint.
- ■ **Calcaneum** – this is known as the heel bone and is the largest and strongest bone of the foot.
- ■ **Cuboid** – this bone is situated between the fourth and fifth metatarsals and the calcaneum. The position of this bone is important in reflexology as it is the demarcation line for the waist.
- ■ **Cuneiforms** – there are three cuneiform bones (outer, medial and inner). All cuneiform bones are located between the navicular bone and the first three metatarsals.
- ■ **Navicular** – this bone is located between the talus bone and the three cuneiforms.

- **Metatarsals** – there are five metatarsals in each foot and they articulate proximally with the cuboid and cuneiforms and distally with the phalanges.
- **Phalanges** – these are the toe bones; there are three in each toe and two in the big toe.

Arches of the foot

In order to provide the spring in the step for walking, running and jumping, the feet must be able to absorb shock. In order to accomplish this, the foot has a system of arches which prevent the plantar surface of the foot (the sole) from becoming flat.

- **Medial longitudinal arch** – this is formed by the calcaneum, talus, navicular, cuneiforms and the medial three metatarsals.
- **Lateral longitudinal arch** – this is formed by the calcaneum, cuboid and the four or five lateral metatarsals.
- **Transverse arch** – this lies across the base of all the metatarsals and is formed by the tarso-metatarsal joint.

In addition to the above, each foot has 31 joints, over 50 ligaments, over 7000 nerve endings and more than 20 intrinsic muscles.

MAPPING OF THE REFLEXES

In reflexology, the feet are often likened to a mini-map of the body: all organs, glands and body parts are reflected in the feet in an almost identical way to the body. The mapping of reflex areas stems from Eunice Ingham's work which was based on her experiences of how the reflex points on the feet were related to corresponding areas in the body.

> **KEY NOTE** It should be remembered that when looking at reflex charts, there may be variations in the position of the reflexes as they reflect an idealistic representation of the reflexes areas and may be different according to personal experience. Reflexologists should therefore use a chart as a guide but use their own judgement and intuition when working with clients.

Reflexes are found on the soles, tops of the feet and along the inside (**medial**) and outside (**lateral**) parts of the feet. The arrangement of reflexes on the feet is roughly similar to the arrangement of corresponding parts of the body. Areas of the feet which relate clearly to parts of the body are as follows:

- The **toes** represent the **head** and **neck**.
- The **sides of the feet** represent the major parts of the **skeleton** – on the inner side of the foot is the spine reflex and the outer side relates to the hip, knee, elbow, upper arm and shoulder.
- The **ball of the foot** represents the **thoracic area**.
- The **arch of the foot** represents the **abdominal cavity**.
- The **heel** represents the **pelvic** and **reproductive areas**.
- The **top of the foot** represents the **lymphatic circulation**.

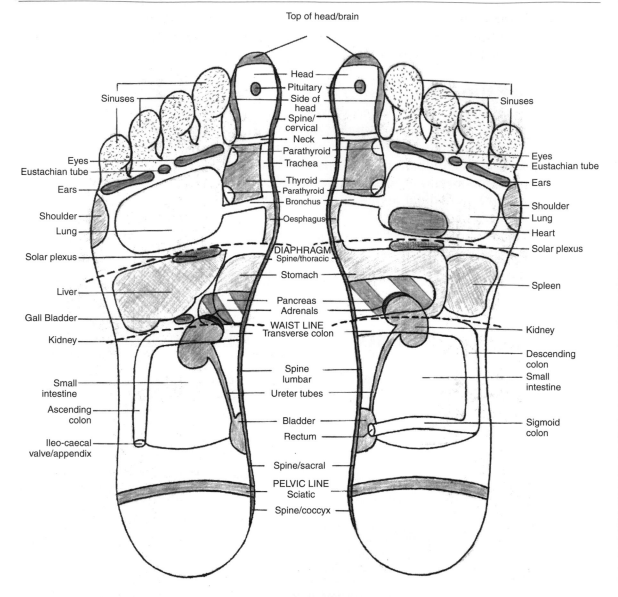

Figure 7.3 Reflex areas of the foot (plantar surface)

Reflexes Associated with the Nervous System

■ **Head and the brain** – the reflex area relating to the head and brain is found in the big toe of each foot.

■ **Hypothalamus** – the reflex area relating to the hypothalamus is found in both feet on the outer side and top of the big toe.

■ **Pineal** – the reflex area relating to the pineal gland is the same as the hypothalamus.

■ **Solar plexus** – the reflex area relating to the solar plexus is found in both feet just below the point relating to the diaphragm in zones 2 and 3.

- **Sciatic** – the reflex area relating to the sciatic nerve is found in both feet across the pad of heel about one-third of the way down. This reflex area also extends up the back of the ankle.

Reflexes Associated with the Endocrine System

- **Pituitary** – the reflex area relating to the pituitary gland is found on the bottom of both feet in the centre of the big toe (where the whorl of the toe print converges into the central point). Usually this reflex area is off-centre, located towards the inner side of the big toe.
- **Thyroid** – the reflex area relating to the thyroid gland is found in both feet over the ball of the big toe.
- **Parathyroids** – the reflex area relating to the parathyroid glands are found in both feet on the lateral side of the thyroid reflex over the ball of the big toe. An upper and a lower reflex is found in both feet, making up the four glands.
- **Adrenals** – the reflex area relating to the adrenal glands is found on the soles of both feet on top of the kidney reflex.

Special Senses Reflexes

- **Eyes** – the reflex area for the eyes is found in both feet on the sole of the foot just below the second and third toes.
- **Ears** – the reflex area for the ears is found in both feet on the sole of the foot just below the fourth and fifth toes.

Reflexes Associated with the Skeletal System

- **Face** – the reflex area for the face is located in both feet on the front of the big toe.
- **Teeth** – the reflexes for the teeth are found in both feet on the fronts of the toes below the nail.
- **Neck** – the reflex for the neck is located in both feet at the base of the big toes where it joints the foot (the back of the neck is represented on the sole of the foot and the front of the neck on top of the foot).
- **Spine** – this reflex is located along the medial side of both feet following the medial longitudinal arch of the foot (the cervical vertebrae are represented from the base of the big toenail down to the base of the big toe, the thoracic spine down to the waist level, the lumbar spine below the waist, and leading back to the heel are the sacrum and coccyx).
- **Hip** – the reflex area relating to the hip is found on both feet on the lateral side of the foot just in front of the heel and behind the knee reflex.
- **Sacro-iliac joint** – the reflex area relating to the sacro-iliac joint is found in both feet in a small indentation on the top of the foot in front of the lateral ankle bone in line with the fourth toe.
- **Shoulder** – the reflex area relating to the shoulder is found in both feet around the base of the little toe on the sole of the foot and on the top of the foot.
- **Upper arm** – the reflex area relating to the arm extends along the lateral side of both feet extending from the shoulder reflex to the elbow reflex.

- **Elbow** – the reflex area relating to the elbow is found on the lateral side of both feet about half way down the lateral side of the foot over a slight bony projection.
- **Knee** – the reflex area relating to the knee is found in both feet on the lateral side extending from the hip area to waist level.
- **Ribs and sternum** – the reflex area relating to the ribs and sternum is located across the top of the foot beneath the toes, above the waist line.

Reflexes Associated with the Muscular System

- **Muscles of the pelvis** – the reflex area relating to the pelvic muscles is on both feet in the area below the lateral ankle bone.

Reflexes Associated with the Respiratory System

- **Sinuses** – the reflex area relating to the sinuses is found in both feet up the backs and the sides of the toes.
- **Eustachian tube** – the reflex area relating to the eustachian tube is found on the sole of both feet in the web of skin in-between the third and fourth toe.
- **Trachea and bronchi** – the reflex area relating to the trachea is found in both feet on the medial side of the foot, leading down from the big toe and the trachea leads across to the plantar surface of the foot into the lung reflex.
- **Lungs** – the reflex area relating to the lungs is found in both feet over the ball of the foot below the second, third, fourth and fifth toes.
- **Diaphragm** – the reflex area relating to the diaphragm is found across the soles of both feet, just below the ball of the foot.

Reflexes Associated with the Circulatory System

- **Heart** – the reflex area relating to the heart is found on the sole of the left foot just above the level of the diaphragm, across the lower part of the ball of the left foot in zones 2 and 3.

Reflexes Associated with the Digestive System

- **Stomach** – the reflex area relating to the stomach is found on the sole of both feet below the level of the diaphragm and above the waist. In the right foot, the pancreas reflex is represented in zones 1 and 2. In the left foot, the pancreas reflex is represented in zones 1 and 3.
- **Pancreas** – the reflex area relating to the pancreas is found in the sole of both feet in the area between the diaphragm and the waist line. In the right foot, the pancreas reflex is represented in zones 1 and 2. In the left foot, the pancreas reflex is represented in zones 1, 2 and 3.
- **Liver** – the reflex area relating to the liver is found on sole of the right foot only and lies in between the diaphragm line and the waist line in zones 3 to 5.
- **Gall bladder** –the reflex area relating to the gall bladder is found on the sole of the right foot only in zone 3 just above the level of the waist line.

- **Small intestine** – the reflex area relating to the small intestine is found on the sole of both feet below the waist level and above the pelvic line extending across zones 1 to 4.
- **Ileo-caecal valve** – the reflex area relating to the ileo-caecal valve is found on the sole of the right foot only just above the pelvic line in zone 4.
- **Appendix** – the reflex area relating to the appendix lies immediately above the ileo-caecal valve.
- **Large intestine/colon** – the reflex areas relating to the large intestine are found in the soles of both feet.
- **Large intestine (in the right foot)**
  The caecum reflex area is found just above the level of the pelvis in zones 4 and 5.
  The ascending colon reflex leads from the caecum reflex up to the waist level.
  The transverse colon reflex extends at the waist level across all five zones.
- **Large intestine (in the left foot)**
  The transverse colon reflex extends at the waist level across all five zones.
  The descending colon reflex extends from the waist line/transverse colon down zones 4 and 5 to a level just above the pelvic line.
  The sigmoid colon reflex continues across from the bottom of the descending colon across to the **rectum** in zone 1.

Reflexology Associated with the Urinary System

- **Kidney** – the reflex area relating to the kidney is found on the sole of both feet at waist level in zones 2 and 3.
- **Bladder** – the reflex area relating to the bladder is found on the medial side of both feet in close proximity to the reflex area for the lumbar spine.

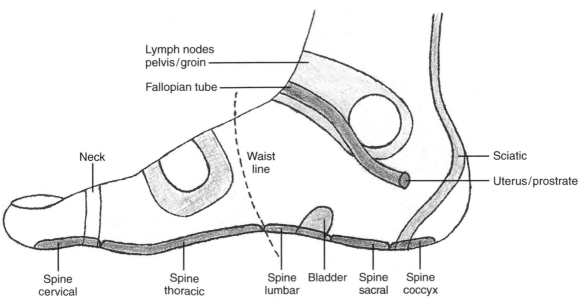

Figure 7.4 Reflex areas of the foot (medial border)

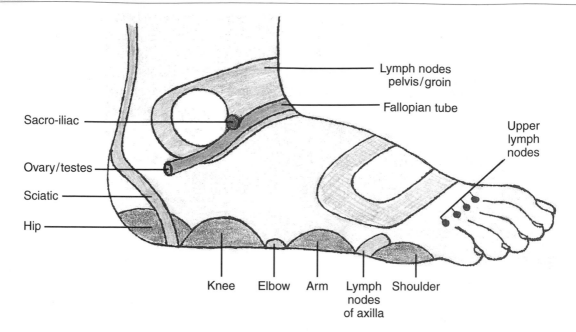

Figure 7.5 Reflex areas of the foot (lateral border)

■ **Ureter** – the reflex area relating to the ureter tube is found on the soles of both feet extending from the bladder to the kidney reflex.

Reflexes Associated with the Female Reproductive System

■ **Ovary** – the reflex area relating to the ovary is found on the medial border of both feet half way between the tip of the lateral ankle bone and the back of the heel.

■ **Uterus** – the reflex area relating to the uterus is found on the medial side of both feet half way between the tip of the medial ankle bone and the back of the heel.

■ **Fallopian tubes** – the reflex area relating to the fallopian tubes is found in both feet joining the reflexes of the ovary and uterus over the top of the foot and in front of the ankle bones.

Reflexes Associated with the Male Reproductive System

■ **Testis** – reflex area relating to the testis is found on the medial border of both feet half way between the tip of the lateral ankle bone and the back of the heel.

■ **Prostate** – the reflex area relating to the prostate is found on the medial side of both feet half way between the tip of the medial ankle bone and the back of the heel.

■ **Vas deferens** – the reflex area relating to the vas deferens is found in both feet joining the reflexes of the testis and prostate over the top of the foot and in front of the ankle bones.

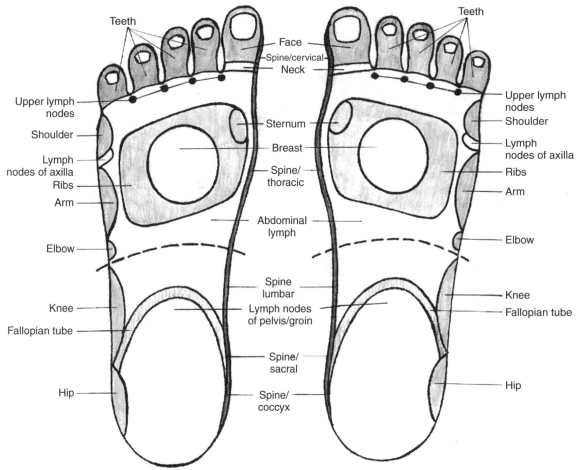

Figure 7.6 Reflex areas of the foot (dorsal surface)

Reflexes Associated with the Lymphatic System

- **Spleen** – the reflex area relating to the spleen is only found on the sole of the left foot beneath the diaphragm and beneath the waist in zones 4 and 5.
- **Thymus** –the reflex area relating to the thymus is found on the soles of both feet over the medial half of the ball of the big toe.
- **Pelvic lymph** – the reflex area relating to the pelvic lymph is on both feet around the across the top of both the medial and lateral ankle bones.
- **Abdominal lymph** – the reflex area relating to abdominal lymph is found in both feet leading from in front of the ankles down in between the metatarsals down to the upper lymph nodes.
- **Axillary lymph** – the reflex area relating to the axillary lymph is found on the top of both feet just below the reflex area for the shoulder.
- **Upper lymph nodes** – the reflex area relating to the upper lymph nodes is found on top of both feet just beneath the toes.
- **Breast** – the reflex area relating to the breast on top of both feet just above waist level in zones 2, 3 and 4.

CAUTIONS AND CONTRA-INDICATIONS FOR REFLEXOLOGY

In general, reflexology is a very safe, natural therapy and there are only a few instances when it would be inadvisable to apply the treatment.

In certain cases it may be necessary to refer the client to their GP before treatment is applied. Where possible, treatment should be adapted to suit the client's conditions and needs.

> **KEY NOTE** In most cases, the contra-indications listed are not generalised enough to prohibit treatment, but should be treated as cautionary. It is, therefore, important for practitioners of reflexology to be aware of the limitations of the treatment and to know when to exercise caution and when to refer the client to their GP.

- **Contagious diseases and illnesses** – due to the risk of spreading infection throughout the body, it is inadvisable to offer reflexology treatment during the acute stages of illness or disease. Treatment should also be avoided in the case of a client suffering from an acute fever.
- **Severe circulatory disorders** – in the case of conditions such as thrombosis and embolism it is advisable to seek medical clearance before treating, due to the theoretical risk that an increase in circulation may move a clot to another part of the body (heart, brain, lungs).
- **Heart conditions** – care should be taken in the case of a severe heart condition to avoid over stimulation. This may overburden the heart and increase the risk of thrombosis or embolism. GP referral is advised.
- **Diabetes** – special care is advised in the case of a diabetic client. They may have neuropathy (decreased or altered sensation), in which case the therapist would monitor the pressure. In most cases the pressure would be lighter. It is also advisable to inform the client's GP in order that their insulin levels may be monitored in response to the reflexology treatment.
- **High blood pressure** – it is advisable to liaise with the client's GP, even if the client is on prescribed medication, due to their susceptibility to form clots. Clients who take anti-hypertensive drugs may be prone to postural hypotension and may experience a feeling of dizziness upon rising. In most cases, as the treatment can help to lower blood pressure, reflexology is very beneficial.
- **Low blood pressure** – care should be taken to help clients upon standing to avoid falls, due to dizziness.
- **Epilepsy** – due to the complexity of this condition, it is advisable to seek the GP's advice regarding the client's suitability for treatment. It has not been proven that reflexology could provoke a convulsion, but caution is advised.
- **Potentially fatal conditions** – in the case of any potentially serious condition, such

as cancer, medical clearance should be sought. There is a risk of certain types of cancer being spread via the lymphatic system and therefore caution is advised. Reflexology has, however, been proven to be a valuable adjunct to the medical treatment of cancer in terms of palliative health care. It supports clients and helps them to cope with their condition.

- **Recent fractures** – if the foot area is affected by a fracture, treatment may be administered to the hands instead.
- **Foot infections** – conditions such as athletes foot and verrucas may be treated as localised contra-indications. Treatment may be administered to the hands instead, until the infection has cleared.
- **Injured, swollen areas and recent haemorrhaging** – care should be taken to avoid any acute injuries in order to avoid discomfort and the risk of exacerbating the condition. In the case of older injuries, reflexology may help to reduce swelling and adhesions.
- **Varicose veins, ulcers and phlebitis** – these should be treated as localised contra-indications, and if severe the client should be referred to their GP.

Special Considerations

- **Osteoporosis** – special care should be taken with the pressure applied, due to the lack of bone density.
- **Painful joints and arthritis** – care should be taken when manipulating acutely inflamed joints. A lighter pressure may be needed.
- **Medication** – caution is advised in the case of clients taking heavy dosages of drugs. This could affect their response to the reflexology treatment, making it stronger due to the increased elimination of the drugs from the bloodstream. Alternatively, the response may be subdued. Seek medical advice if you are unsure about a condition or the potential effects or side effects of the medication.
- **Pregnancy** – pregnancy is not an illness. Many women derive great benefit from the effects of reflexology during pregnancy. In the case of a client with a history of unstable pregnancies, it would be advisable to avoid treatment in the first trimester of the pregnancy. Provided the pregnancy was uncomplicated, later on a lighter and relaxing treatment may be offered.

CLIENT CONSULTATION

Client consultation should always be the first stage of any reflexology treatment. It is required to provide the practitioner with a better understanding of the client's health. The client's medical history may provide information about any imbalance that is detected by the practitioner.

Documenting results and progress is essential for mapping a client's response to treatment and to evaluate patterns that may emerge. On page 168 is an example of a reflexology consultation form.

REFLEXOLOGY CONSULTATION FORM

Client Note

The following information is required for your safety and to benefit your health. Whilst reflexology is a very safe treatment, there are certain conditions which may require special attention. The following information will be treated in the strictest of confidence. It may be necessary for you to consult your GP before treatment can be given..

Date of initial consultation: _____   Client ref. No. _____

Personal Details

Name: _____   Title: Mr/Mrs/Miss/Ms/Other

Address: _____

_____

Telephone Number Daytime: _____   Evening: _____

Date of Birth: _____   Occupation:_____

Medical details

Do you have/have you ever suffered with any of the following conditions?
(Please give dates and details)

			Dates and details
Acne	Y	N	_____
Allergies	Y	N	_____
Dermatitis	Y	N	_____
Eczema	Y	N	_____
Psoriasis	Y	N	_____
Scabies	Y	N	_____
Athletes foot	Y	N	_____
Verucca	Y	N	_____
Other	Y	N	_____

Circulatory Disorders

			Dates and details
Heart condition	Y	N	_____
High or low blood pressure	Y	N	_____
Oedema	Y	N	_____
Thrombosis or embolism	Y	N	_____
Varicose veins	Y	N	_____
Chilblains	Y	N	_____
Recent haemorrhage	Y	N	_____
Other	Y	N	_____

Musculo-Skeletal Disorders

Dates and details

Arthritis	Y	N	_____
Muscular aches and pains	Y	N	_____
Rheumatism	Y	N	_____
Fractures	Y	N	_____
Strains or sprains	Y	N	_____
Other	Y	N	_____

Respiratory Problems

Dates and details

Allergies (i.e. hayfever)	Y	N	_____
Asthma	Y	N	_____
Bronchitis	Y	N	_____
Breathing difficulties	Y	N	_____
Throat infections	Y	N	_____
Sinusitis	Y	N	_____
Colds / Flu	Y	N	_____
Other	Y	N	_____

Digestive Problems

Dates and details

Constipation	Y	N	_____
Indigestion	Y	N	_____
Colitis	Y	N	_____
Candida	Y	N	_____
Irritable bowel syndrome	Y	N	_____
Other	Y	N	_____

Circulatory Disorders

Dates and details

Heart condition	Y	N	_____
High or low blood pressure	Y	N	_____
Oedema	Y	N	_____
Thrombosis or embolism	Y	N	_____
Varicose veins	Y	N	_____
Chilblains	Y	N	_____
Recent haemorrhage	Y	N	_____
Other	Y	N	_____

Musculo-Skeletal Disorders

Dates and details

Arthritis	Y	N	_____
Muscular aches and pains	Y	N	_____
Rheumatism	Y	N	_____
Fractures	Y	N	_____
Strains or sprains	Y	N	_____
Other	Y	N	_____

Respiratory Problems

Dates and details

Allergies (i.e. hayfever)	Y	N	_____
Asthma	Y	N	_____
Bronchitis	Y	N	_____
Breathing difficulties	Y	N	_____
Throat infections	Y	N	_____
Sinusitis	Y	N	_____
Colds / Flu	Y	N	_____
Other	Y	N	_____

Digestive Problems

Dates and details

Constipation	Y	N	_____
Indigestion	Y	N	_____
Colitis	Y	N	_____
Candida	Y	N	_____
Irritable bowel syndrome	Y	N	_____
Other	Y	N	_____

Urinary Problems

Dates and details

Cystitis	Y	N	_____
Thrush	Y	N	_____
Other	Y	N	_____

Nervous or Stress-related problems

Dates and details

Any nervous dysfunction	Y	N	_____
Epilepsy	Y	N	_____
Anxiety	Y	N	_____
Depression	Y	N	_____
Headaches	Y	N	_____

Migraine	Y	N	_____
Insomnia	Y	N	_____
Nervous tension	Y	N	_____
Other	Y	N	_____

Endocrine Disorders

Dates and details

Diabetes	Y	N	_____
Thyroid Problems	Y	N	_____

Other Health-Related Information

Dates and details

Have you had a recent operation?	Y	N	_____
Have you had a potentially fatal or terminal condition?	Y	N	_____

Female Clients

Dates and details

Is it possible that you may be pregnant?	Y	N	_____
Any complications with the pregnancy?	Y	N	_____
Do you have pre-menstrual tension?	Y	N	_____
Menopausal problems?	Y	N	_____
Problems with periods?	Y	N	_____
Other?	Y	N	_____

Are there any other conditions you have, which may affect the proposed treatment?
Y ( )   N ( )

Details _____

_____

Are you currently taking any medication? Y ( )   N ( )

Details (including dosages) _____

_____

Section for use by therapist
GP referral required: Yes ( )   No ( )
Clearance form sent: Yes ( )   No ( )   Date:_____
Clearance form received: Yes ( )   No ( )   Date:_____

Name of Doctor: _____   Surgery: _____

Address: _____

_____

Telephone Number: _____

Lifestyle

Is your general health/immunity: Good ( ) Average ( )   Poor ( )

Are your stress levels: High ( ) Medium ( )   Low ( )

Are your energy levels: High ( ) Medium ( )   Low ( )

Typical daily diet: _____

Number of glasses of water consumed daily: _____

Number of cups of tea/coffee per day: _____

Vitamins/minerals taken:_____

Typical weekly alcohol consumption: _____

Do you smoke: Y ( ) N ( ) if yes how many daily? _____

Do you find time for relaxation/hobbies: Y ( )   N ( )

Details: _____

_____

Have you had reflexology or any other complementary therapy treatment before?

(please state when and the success obtained) _____

_____

Client Declaration

I declare that the information I have given is correct and as far as I am aware, I can undertake treatments without any adverse effects.

I have been fully informed about contra-indications and am therefore willing to proceed
with treatment.

I understand that Reflexology does not substitute medical treatment.

Client's signature: _____   Date: _____

Therapist's signature: _____   Date: _____

RECORD-KEEPING AND TREATMENT-PLANNING FOR REFLEXOLOGY

Treatment-planning is an essential part of a reflexology treatment: the aim is to tailor an individual programme to suit the client's needs. A treatment plan for reflexology will typically include the following information:

- the date of treatment
- feedback from any previous treatment, noting the client's response and any improvements or changes in their condition (if applicable)
- any new information about the client's condition which is needed to update the original consultation form
- the treatment objectives and any specific client needs
- an outline of the proposed treatment, to include treatment strategy (frequency of treatments, length of treatment and cost).

In addition to the above information, it is important for a reflexologist to record the following:

- the type of medium used for foot massage
- a manual and visual analysis of the client's reflexes and the condition of the imbalances presented (it may be helpful to use terms of reference such as crunchy, crystalline, hard, lumpy, puffy to describe the congestion of the reflexes – see page 182 – terms such as tender, sharp, painful, bruised, tingly etc can be used to indicate what the client felt)
- observations of the condition of the client's feet (noting skin temperature, any areas of hard skin or cracks in the skin, tension or puffiness)
- any additional work carried out
- any known contra-actions, their effects on the client and the advice given
- after care advice given
- home care advice given, along with any recommendations for home treatment
- outcome and evaluation of the treatment.

EQUIPMENT FOR REFLEXOLOGY TREATMENT

The beauty of reflexology is that it may be practised virtually anywhere. Treatment may be offered to a client positioned on a treatment couch, in a reclining chair, or with the feet on a foot stool designed for reflexology, such as the Portaped.

There are a few other resources needed for reflexology which include:

- bolsters and cushions to offer support to the head, neck, back, knees and ankles
- a blanket (in case the client feels cold during the treatment)
- clean towels and disposable tissues to cover the work area
- some form of lubricant (see note below), preferably with a pump dispenser or in a canister to avoid contamination
- foot cleanser, to cleanse the client's feet prior to treatment
- a small bin to dispose of any used materials.

> **KEY NOTE** The use of lubricants in reflexology is a controversial issue: some practitioners advocate the use of a lubricant; others prefer to work without one. If choosing to use a lubricant, it is important that the practitioner avoids using one which inhibits their movements or interferes with their tactile analysis of the reflexes.
>
> A very light application of cream or powder (corn starch or Vita Fons) is recommended. This enables the reflexologist to work freely, but without the true texture of the reflexes being masked by the medium.

PREPARATION FOR A REFLEXOLOGY TREATMENT

Preparation of the Therapist

■ Ensure nails are short, clean and unvarnished.
■ Present a professional image with the correct workwear.
■ Tie hair back if long.
■ Ensure good personal hygiene.
■ The treatment room should be hygienically clean with good ventilation.
■ Ensure all materials needed for the treatment are close to hand.
■ Wash hands before and after the treatment.

Preparation of the Client for a Reflexology Treatment

■ Carry out a client consultation to establish the client's suitability for treatment and the objectives of the treatment.
■ Cleanse the client's feet or offer bowl of warm water to soak the feet in – check the feet for any infectious disorders.
■ Help the client onto the couch, with the use of a foot stool if necessary.
■ Position the client comfortably, with supports for the head, back, ankles and knees (some clients like to lie flat, but it is preferable for the client to be in a semi-reclined position, in order that their facial expressions may be observed).

SUGGESTED REFLEXOLOGY TREATMENT METHOD

There are many different methods for reflexology practice. The purpose of this book is therefore not to show a definitive way to apply treatment. Some reflexologists prefer to work the reflexes of one foot before proceeding to the other, whilst others prefer to work each foot systematically.

Whatever method of reflexology is employed, it is important to ensure that each reflex area is covered and that the treatment is adapted to suit the needs of the individual client. A reflexology session generally commences with some relaxation techniques; the reflexes will be more accessible to the reflexologist if the client is relaxed and if the tissue is pliable.

Relaxation techniques

The aim of a reflexology treatment is to offer deep relaxation, which will assist the nervous system to obtain a state of balance and which encourages the body to recover from stress. Relaxation exercises are used **before** a reflexology treatment in order to:

- relax the client and prepare them for the treatment
- release tension by loosening up the feet
- help to encourage deep breathing
- to maximise the effects of the reflexology treatment.

During a reflexology treatment similar exercises are used to:

- calm and soothe an area of discomfort
- encourage relaxation if the client is particularly tense.

After a reflexology treatment exercises can:

- Soothe and relax the client at the end of the treatment

Examples of relaxation techniques which may be used, during or after reflexology include:

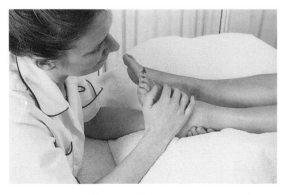

Figure 7.8 Lower back release

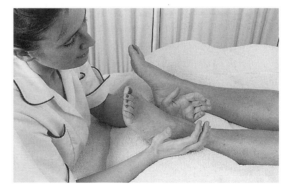

Figure 7.9 Ankle loosening

Lower back release – with one hand supporting under the back of the ankle and one hand on top of the ankle perform a gentle traction movement by drawing the client's foot back towards you. This helps to loosen the hips and pelvic muscles. *Repeat 3 or 4 times on one foot and then repeat on the other.*

Ankle loosening – with the heel of both hands inserted under the outer malleoli bones perform a gentle rocking movement up and down to loosen up the ankle joint (you will know if this movement is performed correctly as the foot will move from side to side) *Repeat several times until ankle joint starts to loosen*

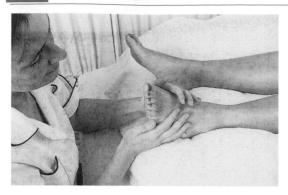

Figure 7.10 Foot loosening

Foot loosening – shape your hands round the lateral part of the client's foot and perform a brisk rocking movement up and down the foot. This technique is very effective for warming the foot and helping to increase the circulation. *Repeat several times until the foot feels looser and then repeat on the other foot*

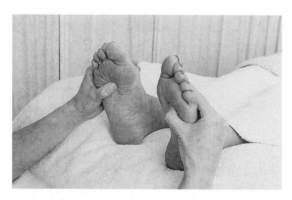

Figure 7.12 Solar plexus breathing

Solar plexus breathing – insert both thumbs into the solar plexus reflex of each of the client's feet. Ask the client to take a deep breath in through the nose and as they breathe in push the foot up and outwards. As they breathe out release the thumb and return the feet to their original position. *Repeat 3 or 4 times.*

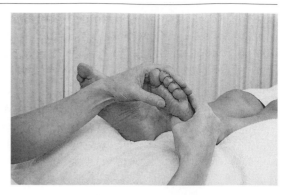

Figure 7.11 Tension reliever

Tension Reliever – perform thumb walking across the diaphragm reflex area, whilst supporting the top of the foot with the other hand. As the thumb presses into the diaphragm reflex pull the toes down as if pressing down onto the diaphragm and then release the thumb and the toes. Continue this motion across the whole of the diaphragm reflex one way and change hands to repeat the other way. *Repeat this several times across the back until the tension in the foot is released.*

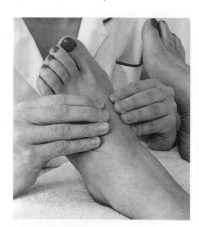

Figure 7.13 Drainage across the top of the foot

Drainage across the top of the foot – draw the fingers of one hand across the top of the foot (the area below the toes) from big toe out towards the little toe, whilst keeping a supporting hand at the medial side of the foot. Repeat further down across the foot until all the lymphatic channels of the top of the foot have been covered.

The relaxation techniques give the reflexologist an idea of the tensions held in the feet. Other observations may also be made, such as the temperature and texture of the feet, which may be significant indicators of the imbalances present. The solar plexus reflex is often the key to relaxation.

> **KEY NOTE** The solar plexus is a very large nerve plexus located behind the stomach and in front of the diaphragm. It is often referred to as the 'abdominal or feeling brain' as it is the centre for our feeling and emotions.
>
> In reflexology, the solar plexus is an incredibly powerful reflex. It effectively calms and releases pent-up tension, regulates breathing and induces a state of deep relaxation.
>
> Any resistance or tightness of this reflex area is indicative of anxiety, tension and stress. Calming this reflex can be extremely beneficial and can restore a sense of emotional balance.

REFLEXOLOGY TECHNIQUE

The basic reflexology technique is one of compression and relaxation. The compression technique may be applied with either the thumbs or the fingers. The thumbs are generally used on the areas of the feet with thicker padding, such as the plantar surface and the fingers are generally used on the dorsum of the foot where there is less padding.

The technique is applied with the inside (medial) edge of the thumb, or finger. It consists of bending and unbending the digit at the first phalangeal joint, so that the thumb or finger takes small steps along the foot (this is called the **compression phase** or thumb or finger walking). It is the bending movement of the first joint that moves the thumb forwards, so that it may be pushed specifically and systematically into each reflex point.

In order to move onto the next reflex point, the thumb is moved off the current point by easing back slightly and then easing forwards onto the next point (the **relaxation phase**).

It is thought that reflex points on the feet and hands are approximately one-sixteenth of an inch apart. Therefore, it is important for the practitioner to take small steps in order to avoid missing any areas in need of help.

> **KEY NOTE** It is important for the practitioner to develop a slow to moderate rhythm of compression and relaxation. This helps to encourage the parasympathetic nervous system to facilitate rest, repair and the restoration of energy in the body.

'Walking' over the reflex points with the thumbs and fingers gives the practitioner an opportunity to assess the imbalances. By stimulating the relevant points, the practitioner may help to ease tension, dissolves blockages and boost the circulation of energy to all the organs and parts of the body to encourage healing.

It is important, when practising thumb or finger walking, that the client's foot or hand is held by the therapist in their other hand, in order to provide support and leverage for the movements. It is important for the practitioner to be able to switch hands freely to work the tender reflexes in different directions (up and down, from left to right and from right to left). Working across a reflex area one way may produce no sensitivity and yet working from another direction may prove to be very sensitive.

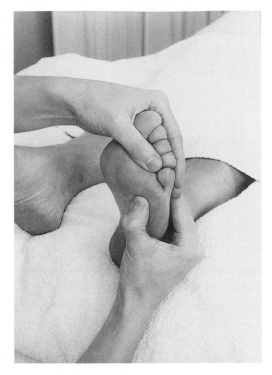

Figure 7.14 Supporting the foot correctly

Other Reflexology Techniques

In reflexology, the basic compression technique is designed for walking of the reflexes along the pathways of all zones. There are additional techniques that may also be used to work the reflexes.

Rotating or Pivoting on a Point

This technique involves increasing the pressure applied by the thumb or finger, by rotating or reflexing the foot onto the reflex area. This is a valuable technique for working on very tender reflexes, as it helps to shift the pressure and discomfort from the affected areas.

Hook-in and Back-up Technique

This is a specific technique used to access small and deep-seated reflexes (such as the pituitary, pineal and hypothalamus, ileo-caecal valve, appendix and sigmoid colon). These areas may not be stimulated sufficiently by the basic compression technique.

The technique involves flexing the first joint of the thumb and exerting pressing with the inside corner of the thumb. Once the thumb is placed on a reflex point on the foot, it is hooked in by sinking into the point. Then, whilst maintaining the pressure, the thumb is pulled back across the point (hence 'backing-up').

Duration and Frequency of Treatment

The duration of a reflexology treatment will depend on the client's condition. The first treatment session usually takes a little longer, due to the initial consultation, exploration of the medical history and the discussion of a treatment plan or strategy. A reflexology treatment usually takes approximately 1 hour and it may consist of:

- 5 minutes to ascertain the client's current state of health and to go over the treatment plan
- 5 minutes preliminary relaxation techniques
- 40 minutes reflexology treatment
- 5 minutes concluding massage techniques
- 5 minutes rest before leaving.

The frequency of treatment depends on the client's condition, and other resources such as time and money. A client with a chronic, well-established condition is likely to need more frequent treatment than a client with a more acute problem. An important consideration is that there needs to be a balance between having enough treatment to see results and allowing enough time to elapse in order for the body to heal.

If a client presents with a specific problem, it is good practice to advise a course of six to 12 treatments, initially attending twice a week and then once a week thereafter. It is important to stress to the client that, by attending more frequently to start with, they will feel a faster improvement in their health as the effects of the treatment are cumulative.

It is inadvisable to apply a full treatment more than twice weekly as this may prove to be too taxing for the client. However, some clients may need daily treatment of certain specific reflex areas in order to help with pain relief. Clients may be shown reflex areas to work on their own hands. This is useful back-up in between treatments with a reflexologist.

> **KEY NOTE** It is important to stress to clients that the positive effects of reflexology are dependent on regular application, but also by their own responsiveness to the treatment.

Treating a Specific Area

When considering how long to work an individual area with reflexology, give thought to the client's tolerance and their individual condition. Reflexes need to have sufficient stimulus in order to effect a response. However, this should not be to the point of causing severe discomfort to the client. Depending on the tolerance levels of the client, individual reflex areas may be worked for up to a minute. If the area presents with a multitude of imbalances, the practitioner should use relaxation techniques and go back to give the area additional work at a later stage in the treatment.

ADAPTATIONS OF REFLEXOLOGY TREATMENT

It is important that reflexology treatments are adapted to suit the individual needs of a client. The reflexology treatment should always be approached in an holistic way by attending to all the main reflex areas. Additional treatment or specific techniques may also be applied to treat certain areas presenting imbalance and congestion.

> **KEY NOTE** Clients will inevitably present with different clinical conditions. It is important for the reflexologist to be aware of specific disorders and how they may affect a client's condition.
>
> Specific reflexology books offer information on specific disorders relating to specific systems of the body. Reflexologists are encouraged to carry out as much research as possible in order to gain an insight into which reflexes could be worked to aid a particular client's recovery. The introductory pathology section in this book (pages 13-41) may also serve as a guide to presenting symptoms and how the treatment may be adapted.

Associated or Helper Areas

These are reflex areas that may be used to help relieve the congestion in affected areas in order to increase the effectiveness of the reflexology treatment. For instance, a client presenting for treatment with a tension headache may require additional work to be carried out to the helper reflex areas of the neck, shoulders, upper arms and back, depending on the cause of the headache. It is important to assess each client's conditions and imbalances in an holistic way, in order that cause is addressed and not just the symptoms.

Referral Areas

These are a useful adjunct to reflexology. They allow the practitioner to swap treatment for one area of the body to an alternate area. This can be done if the two parts have an anatomical relationship to one another. Referral areas or zone-related areas are especially useful in the case of an injury or infected area that may not be treated. They may also be used in addition to the referral areas to enhance the effectiveness of the treatment.

> Zone-related areas are as follows:
> - the hand with the foot
> - the hip with the shoulder
> - the elbow with the knee
> - the ankle with the wrist
> - the upper thigh with the upper arm
> - the lower leg with the forearm.

Disabled clients

Disabled clients should be treated with sensitivity and respect. Depending on the nature of their disability, they may have reflexology in a wheelchair or on a treatment couch. The client's comfort is paramount and the practitioner must have sufficient access to the feet. Disabled clients should be treated no differently than another client; the practitioner should be aware of the client's condition to be able to assess how reflexology may help. Shorter, more frequent sessions may be advisable, and the disabled client and their carer may be shown reflex areas to work at home.

Elderly clients

Important considerations when treating elderly clients include the following:

- The application of pressure should be modified as there may be a lack of bone density. Skin may also be thinner and weaker, and bruising may occur.
- Elderly clients may be unable to give adequate feedback due to insensitivity and/or medication being taken.
- The client's range of motion may be limited; always work within the client's comfortable range of movement, particularly when mobilising the ankle and foot.
- If the client's condition is chronic, it may be advisable to apply shorter treatments more frequently.
- Clients may tire more easily. They may have a stronger reaction to the treatment, due to the accumulation of a lifetime of imbalances.

Pregnant Clients

Important considerations when offering a reflexology treatment to a pregnant client include the following:

- Avoid treatment in the first trimester of the pregnancy until the pregnancy is established.
- If there have been previous complications, such as miscarriage, obtain advice from the client's GP.
- Avoid applying pressure to the reproductive reflexes, and concentrate on relaxation techniques instead.
- Give a shorter session.
- Teach the client how to work reflexes on their hands so that either they or their partner may use the technique to ease discomfort in the later stages of pregnancy. Swollen ankles and backache can be helped in this way. Partners may also be taught reflexes to give help during childbirth which may aid pain relief.

Children

Guidelines for using reflexology techniques with children include:

- Gain parental consent and the consent of the child before treating.
- Use a lighter pressure, remembering that the bones are soft and still growing.
- Add an element of fun to the treatment by involving the children as much as possible. For instance, techniques may be demonstrated on their favourite teddy.
- Parents may be shown reflex areas to work at home in order to enhance the effectiveness of the treatment.

■ The length of the session should be brief so as not to lose the child's interest and to avoid overworking.

ASSESSING IMBALANCE

To practise reflexology it is important to understand and to be able to interpret imbalances, as they may offer insight into the condition of the corresponding areas. Imbalances may be detected in several ways by the practitioner. They should always be interpreted in light of the client's individual case history:

Visual Assessment

General observations should be made of the appearance of the feet. Clinical signs may indicate an imbalance within the system. Significant factors should be noted and evaluated, such as any areas of hard skin, oedema, swelling and puffiness, skin texture and colour, any areas of infection.

Tactile Assessment

A reflexologist may be able to interpret signs of imbalance through tactile awareness. Signs of imbalance and that a client's energy may be low include numbness or insensitivity, coldness, dampness or clamminess, tension in the tissues, sponginess in the tissues.

There are several textures that may be felt on a client's feet (or hands):
■ **Crystalline** – this texture feels like grains of sand and indicates congested areas of tissue and areas of imbalance. This texture usually indicates an acute condition and may feel like a very sharp pain to the client.
■ **Lumpy** – this type of reflex is usually undulating to the touch and can indicate a chronic condition, especially if the client's vitality is low. The pain from this type of textured reflex may not feel sharp, but may feel bruised and heavy to the touch.
■ **Spongy** – this type of texture usually indicates a chronic condition, with low vitality and lymphatic stasis.

The Client's Response

The client may experience tenderness, soreness and pain as the reflexes areas are worked.

> **KEY NOTE** It is important to note that tenderness and sensitivity in the reflexes may not show until the third or fourth treatment as the area may lack the energy to respond, indicating that the client's vitality is low. It is, therefore, important that the reflexologist is able to interpret the state of the reflexes using touch and does not rely solely on feedback given by the client.

It is also important to consider that tenderness in a reflex area may indicate past, as well as present, trauma. Clients may experience a subdued response due to a lack of vitality or heavy medication.

REACTIONS TO REFLEXOLOGY

In general, reflexology is a pleasurable experience. However, it is prudent to be aware of possible reactions and responses that may occur in order that you can explain them to the client. It is important to remember that no two clients will react in the same way as everyone is unique.

Detoxification is the only true path to restoring health and vitality. It is possible that the body may experience some form of 'healing crisis' as it attempts to heal itself and rid itself of unwanted toxins.

> **KEY NOTE** The degree of reaction following treatment will depend on the degree of imbalance and the parts of the system which are congested. A healing crisis may occur during a reflexology treatment or shortly afterwards. It is essential that the client understands the reaction is a positive sign that the reflexology is working. Conditions may worsen before they get better.

Possible Reactions During a Reflexology Treatment

The following may occur during treatment:

- warmth or coldness in the corresponding area being treated
- changes in facial expression
- visible contraction of the muscles
- signalling of pain
- twitching
- tingling or itchy sensation
- coughing
- sweating and clamminess of the palms of the hands and the soles of the feet
- emotional release of laughter or tears
- sighing deeply or yawning
- movement in the corresponding areas being treated
- headache
- a cold, shivery feeling.

Possible Reactions After a Reflexology Treatment

The following could occur after treatment:

- increased urination
- increased bowel movement, with possible flatulence
- a disturbed sleep pattern (restlessness with vivid dreams)
- an improved sleep pattern (deep and restful)
- cold-like symptoms
- a feeling of extreme lethargy and tiredness
- a temporary outbreak of a condition that has been suppressed
- feverishness
- headache
- increased energy levels
- aches and pains the day after treatment

- elevation of mood
- pain relief
- increased joint mobility
- depression.

EVALUATION OF THE REFLEXOLOGY TREATMENT

Clients should be offered a glass of water after the reflexology session. They should be left to rest for a few minutes before getting up. After the treatment, the reflexologist will want to discuss the client's response. It is essential to know how the client is feeling in order that their treatment plan may be evaluated and reviewed. Clients may wish to discuss the reflexologist's evaluation of the imbalances present and should be encouraged to do so, as it helps involve them in their own progress.

> **KEY NOTE** It is very important for a reflexologist to avoid diagnosing a condition based on the imbalances presented in the reflex areas. This may cause undue concern, and the reflexologist would be giving unqualified advice.
>
> There may not always be a conclusive reason why certain areas are tender or congested. Wherever possible the therapist's findings should be evaluated in line with the client's physical and emotional state at the time of treatment (although imbalances may also relate to past trauma). If there are any areas for concern then the client should be referred to their GP for medical advice.

AFTER CARE ADVICE

The following advice may be given to enhance the effectiveness of the treatment:

- Drink plenty of water over the following few days to assist in the detoxification of the body.
- Have a suitable rest period to facilitate healing.

Part of the client's after care advice may involve making lifestyle changes or changes to the dietary habits. The client may be shown areas of the hands and feet to work for self-help in between professional treatments.

Clients should be encouraged to book a course of treatments or to attend for treatment regularly in order that they may benefit from the cumulative effects of reflexology. Once a client has made significant progress, they should have a maintenance treatment once a month to help keep them in balance.

CHAPTER 8
Indian head massage

INTRODUCTION

Indian head massage is an extremely effective treatment that has evolved from traditional techiques practised in India, as part of a family ritual, for over a thousand years. The treatment is non-invasive: the massage is applied through the clothes and, thus, can be performed anywhere. Indian head massage is an holistic treatment. It works on both a physical and psychological level and the treatment, which is applied to the upper back, shoulders, upper arms, neck, face and scalp, represents a de-stressing programme for the whole body.

Although an extremely popular treatment, conventional massage still harbours a number of barriers for some clients. They may be too embarrassed to remove their clothing or there may be certain constraints in their daily life, such as time. Indian head massage is starting to bridge this gap in the massage market: its strengths lie in the fact that it is quick to apply, it can be carried out anywhere, and the client remains fully clothed. In addition, no special equipment is required to perform it. Although Indian head massage has been in existence in India for many years, it has only recently started to gain popularity in the West.

A BRIEF HISTORY OF INDIAN HEAD MASSAGE

Ayurveda is the world's oldest recorded healing system. The early Ayurvedic texts, dating back nearly 4000 years, feature massage and the principles of holistic treatment. They promoted the belief that health results from the harmony within oneself.

KEY NOTE Massage has been an important feature of Indian family life across the generations. In India, it is customary for babies to be massaged every day from birth and this is continued until they are 3 years old. From the age of 6, they are taught to show love and respect by sharing a massage with family members.

The techniques practised today have evolved from traditional rituals of Indian family grooming. Indian women have been taught by their mothers to use different oils, such as coconut, sesame, olive, almond, herbal oils, buttermilk, mustard oil and henna, on their scalps in order to maintain their hair in beautiful condition.

Indian barbers developed a head massage which was incorporated into their service. This differed from the women's treatment in that it was more invigorating and stimulating, rather than being part of a beautifying ritual. This also has been passed down through the generations from barber father to barber son. In India, head massage is not just performed at home within families but is available on street corners, at the beach and in barbers shops.

Today, Indian head massage has become a stress management programme. The original techniques performed in India have been developed to become Westernised and include massage to areas that are most vulnerable to stress and tension, such as the neck and shoulders.

BENEFITS AND EFFECTS

Indian head massage is an holistic treatment and, therefore, it has many physiological and psychological benefits.

Physical Benefits

Indian head massage can:

- improve blood flow to the head and neck, increasing the distribution of nutrients into the tissues and encouraging healing
- improve lymphatic drainage in the head and neck, increasing the elimination of toxins and waste material from the body
- relieve muscular tension
- relieve physical and emotional stress
- reduce fibrous adhesions and constrictions from tense muscle fibres
- improve joint mobility by unlocking restricted joint movements
- help to improve muscle tone
- help boost the blood supply to the scalp, promoting healthy hair growth
- encourage the supply of blood to the head and the brain, helping to clear the mind
- help to relieve mental and physical strain, increasing productivity
- increase the blood supply to the brain promoting clearer thinking and improved concentration
- promote deep relaxation and can help to induce sleep
- help to relieve eyestrain and tension headaches
- help to relieve congestion in the head (associated with sinusitis, tinnitus)
- improve respiration by encouraging deeper breathing.

Psychological Benefits

This form of massage

- is an antidote to stress, anxiety and depression
- creates a balanced feeling of peace and calm as stagnant energy is released and the energy flow to the body is rebalanced
- refreshes and revitalises the mind and body.

CAUTIONS AND CONTRA-INDICATIONS FOR INDIAN HEAD MASSAGE

In certain cases it may be necessary to refer the client to their GP before treatment is applied. Where possible, treatment should be adapted to suit the client's conditions and needs.

- **High temperature or fever** – this is a contra-indication because of the risk of spreading infection as a result of the increased circulation.
- **Acute infectious disease** – these would be contra-indicated due to the fact that they are highly contagious.
- **Skin or scalp infections** – these may be worsened and spread by the massage. Advise the client to seek advice and treatment from their GP.
- **Recent haemorrhage** – haemorrhaging is excessive bleeding which may be either external or internal. Massage should be avoided due to the risk of blood spillage from the blood vessels.
- **Intoxication** – it is inadvisable to carry out treatment whilst a client is under the influence of alcohol. The increase in blood flow to the head could make them feel dizzy and nauseous.
- **Recent head or neck injury** – it is not advisable to treat clients who have had a recent blow to the head with concussion, or an acute neck injury, such as whiplash. This is due to the risk of exacerbating the condition and increasing the inflammation and pain. However, if there is an old injury, massage may help to reduce scar tissue, decrease pain and increase mobility. Always obtain medical clearance to ensure the client is suitable for treatment.
- **Recent surgery** – depending on the site of the surgery, it may be necessary to obtain medical clearance before carrying out treatment.
- **Severe circulatory disorders and heart conditions** – always obtain medical clearance before treating a client with a severe heart condition or circulatory problem, as the increased circulation from the massage may overburden the heart and can increase the risk of thrombus or embolus.
- **Thrombosis or embolism** – there is a theoretical risk that a blood clot may become detached from its site of formation and be carried to another part of the body. Always refer to the client's GP for advice on the severity of the condition before offering treatment.
- **High blood pressure** – clients with high blood pressure should be referred to their GP prior to Indian head massage, even if they are on prescribed medication, due to their susceptibility to form clots. Clients on anti-hypertensive drugs may be prone to

postural hypotension and may feel light headed and dizzy after treatment. Therapists should advise clients to get up slowly after treatment.

■ **Low blood pressure** – see above cautions under *high blood pressure*.

■ **Dysfunction of the nervous system** – clients with any dysfunction of the nervous system should be referred to their GP before treatment is given. A light, relaxing massage may be indicated in the case of a client with cerebral palsy, multiple sclerosis or parkinsons disease. Massage may help to reduce spasms, involuntary movements, rigidity and stiffness. Always seek medical advice before offering treatment.

■ **Epilepsy** – always refer to the client's GP regarding the type and nature of the client's epilepsy. Caution is advised due to the complexity of this condition and the risk that deep relaxation or over stimulation could provoke a convulsion (although this has not been proven in practice). As some types of epilepsy may be triggered by smells, care should be taken with choice of oils or medium.

■ **Diabetes** – this is a condition that requires medical referral, as clients with diabetes may be prone to arteriosclerosis, high blood pressure and oedema. Pressure should be applied carefully. The client may have some loss of sensory function and may be unable to give accurate feedback. If the client is receiving insulin by injection, care should be taken to avoid massage on recent injection sites (this type of massage usually extends to the arms). Clients should have their medication with them when they attend for treatment, in case of an emergency.

■ **Cancer** – medical clearance should always be sought before massaging a client with cancer. It is unlikely that gentle massage can cause cancer to spread through the stimulation of lymph flow. However, it is important to obtain advice from the consultant or medical team about the type of cancer and the extent of the disease. If massage is indicated, avoid massage over areas of the body receiving radiation therapy, close to tumour sites and areas of skin cancer. Light massage can help the client to relax and it supports the immune system.

■ **Skin disorders** – care should be taken as the condition may be worsened by massage. Some skin conditions such as eczema, dermatitis and psoriasis should be treated as a localised contra-indication. Affected areas may be hypersensitive and the condition may be exacerbated by massage.

■ **Recent scar tissue** – massage should only be applied once the tissue is fully healed and can withstand pressure. Gentle frictions may be applied over healed scar tissue in order to break down adhesions.

■ **Severe bruising, open cuts or abrasions** – these should be treated as localised contra-indications and, if presented in the treatment areas, they should be avoided.

■ **Undiagnosed lumps, bumps and swellings** – the client should be referred to their GP for a diagnosis. Massage may increase the susceptibility to damage in the area by virtue of pressure and motion.

Special Considerations

■ **Allergies** – ensure that any oils or products used do not contain substances to which the client is allergic. Patch tests should be carried out to avoid adverse reactions.

■ **Medication** – certain medications may inhibit or distort the client's response making it difficult for them to give feedback regarding pressure, discomfort and pain. Always check with the client's GP if you are unsure about their medication and its effects.

■ **Migraine** – it is inadvisable to carry out treatment whilst a client is suffering from a migraine. They may feel nauseous, dizzy and could have visual disturbances. However, Indian head massage may help as a preventative treatment, particularly if their migraines are stress-induced.

■ **Pregnancy** – although pregnancy is not strictly a contra-indication, unless there are serious complications, special care should be taken to ensure that a pregnant client is comfortable during the treatment. Therapists should be aware that some women may experience side effects as a result of the pregnancy, such as dizziness and high blood pressure. Pressure and the duration of treatment should be adjusted according to the individual circumstances.

CLIENT CONSULTATION FOR INDIAN HEAD MASSAGE TREATMENT

A consultation for Indian head massage therapy will cover the following areas:

■ the client's medical history and any current medical treatment
■ general state of health
■ lifestyle patterns
■ any presenting problems
■ client declaration and signature.

Therapists should be tactful when explaining any restrictions to the massage treatment or the reasons for a referral to the GP.

An example of an Indian head massage therapy consultation form is given on page 190. See page 10 for a client referral form if required.

INDIAN HEAD MASSAGE CONSULTATION FORM

Client Note

The following information is required for your safety and to benefit your health. Whilst Indian head massage is a very safe treatment, there are certain conditions which may require special attention. The following information will be treated in the strictest of confidence and it may be necessary for you to consult your GP before treatment can be given.

Date of initial consultation: _____   Client ref. No. _____

Personal Details

Name: _____   Title: Mr/Mrs/Miss/Ms/Other

Address: _____

_____

Telephone Number Daytime: _____   Evening: _____

Date of Birth: _____   Occupation: _____

Medical details

Do you have / have you ever suffered from any of the following conditions? (please give dates and details)

			Dates and Details
High temperature or fever	Y	N	_____
Acute infectious disease	Y	N	_____
Skin infections	Y	N	_____
Recent haemorrhage	Y	N	_____
Recent head or neck injury	Y	N	_____
Recent surgery	Y	N	_____
Severe circulatory disorder	Y	N	_____
Heart condition	Y	N	_____
Thrombosis or embolism	Y	N	_____
High or low blood pressure	Y	N	_____
Dysfunction of the nervous system	Y	N	_____
Epilepsy	Y	N	_____
Diabetes	Y	N	_____
A potentially fatal or terminal condition	Y	N	_____
Recent scar tissue	Y	N	_____
Severe bruising, open cuts or abrasions	Y	N	_____
Undiagnosed lumps, bumps or swellings	Y	N	_____
Allergies	Y	N	_____
Migraine or headaches	Y	N	_____
Scalp infection	Y	N	_____

Are you currently under the influence of alcohol   Y   N   _____
or drugs?

Female Clients

Is it possible that you may be pregnant?   Y   N   _____

Are there any other conditions you have, which may affect the proposed treatment?

Y (   ) N (   )

Details _____

_____

Are you currently taking any medication?   Y (   ) N (   )

Details (including dosages) _____

_____

Section for use by therapist

GP referral required: Yes (   )   No (   )

Clearance form sent: Yes (   )   No (   )   Date:_____

Clearance form received: Yes (   )   No (   )   Date:_____

Name of Doctor: _____   Surgery: _____

Address: _____

_____

Telephone Number: _____

Lifestyle

Is your general health and immunity: Good (   )   Average (   )   Poor (   )

Are your stress levels: High (   )   Medium (   )   Low (   )

Are your energy levels: High (   )   Medium (   )   Low (   )

Do you find time for relaxation/hobbies: Y (   )   N (   )

Details: _____

Client Declaration

I declare that the information I have given is correct and, as far as I am aware, I can undertake treatments without any adverse effects. I have been fully informed about contra-
indications and am, therefore, willing to proceed with treatment. I understand that Indian
head massage is not a substitute for medical treatment.

Client's signature: _____   Date: _____

Therapist's signature: _____   Date: _____

TREATMENT-PLANNING AND RECORD-KEEPING FOR INDIAN HEAD MASSAGE

A treatment plan for Indian head massage will typically include the following information:

- the date of treatment
- feedback from any previous treatments (if applicable), noting the client's responses and any changes or improvement in the client's condition
- any new information relating to the client's condition which is required to update the original consultation form
- the treatment objectives and any particular client needs
- an outline plan of the proposed treatment, to include areas for treatment, length and the cost of the treatment.

In addition, it is important to record the following information as part of the client's record of Indian head massage treatments:

- type of oils used (if applicable)
- an assessment of the client's physical state (noting areas of tension, muscular spasms, adhesions, joint mobility, breathing), as well as the client's psychological responses
- any known contra-actions, their effects on the client and the advice given
- after care advice given
- home care advice given, along with any oils or products suggested for use at home
- outcome and general evaluation of the treatment
- recommendations for future treatment.

MASSAGE MOVEMENTS USED IN INDIAN HEAD MASSAGE

The techniques used in Indian head massage are simple and effective; they consist of a combination of traditional Indian techniques and modern techniques. Strong features of the Indian head massage are the deep friction movements, which are performed with the whole of the hand, the heel of the hand or the fingers, and the lighter, rubbing technique using the ball and the heel of the hand.

Effleurage or Smoothing Movements

These are superficial or deep movements performed with the hand or the forearms which lightly increased the circulation, as well as having soothing and calming effects.

Kneading Movements

These are performed using the thumbs, or the whole hand and fingers. Skin and muscular tissue are moved from their position and are squeezed with a firm pressure away from the underlying structure. Then they are released.

These movements can:

- increase the removal of waste products from the tissue
- encourage fresh oxygen and nutrients to be delivered to the tissues
- stretch muscle tissue and fascia
- reduce adhesions and muscular spasms.

Percussion movements

These movements involve quick, striking manipulations which are highly stimulating to the body. The effects are to:

- increase nervous stimulation
- help tone muscles
- revitalise the body.

Vibrations

These movements are shaking or trembling movements which have the following effects:

- When applied lightly, they are soothing. They bring about relaxation and a release of tension.
- When applied more deeply, they have a stimulating effect on the nerves and are refreshing.

Pressures

These movements are applied with the fingers and the thumbs and their general effects are to:

- clear congestion in the nerve pathways
- increase circulation
- restore energy balance to the body.

CHAKRA BALANCING IN INDIAN HEAD MASSAGE

A person's reaction to stress can create imbalances in the mind and body.

> **KEY NOTE** An important part of Indian head massage treatment is the eastern tradition of balancing of the **higher chakras** (The Throat chakra, the Brow chakra or Third eye, and the Crown Chakra). With stress and tension, the chakras lose their ability to synchronise with one another and become unbalanced. By placing the hands along the axis of the higher chakras, energy can be realigned and a sense of balance and harmony can be restored.

For further information on the chakras see page 67.

EQUIPMENT AND MATERIALS FOR INDIAN HEAD MASSAGE

The beauty of Indian head massage lies in its simplicity. It can be performed in an ordinary chair, without the need to purchase expensive equipment. The type of chair best suited to Indian head massage treatments is one with a relatively low back and without arm rests. An important factor for the therapist is the height of the chair; it is preferable for the therapist to work with the client sitting in a chair with adjustable height and back rest. This enables the therapist to use correct body mechanics.

It is important for a therapist practising Indian head massage to have a variety of oils available for optional use on the scalp, and a hand cleanser. The best type of hand cleanser for a mobile, visiting therapist is a dry anti-bacterial cleanser. These are easy and practical to use.

Oils Used in Indian Head Massage

The use of oil is optional when massaging the scalp. Oils such as sesame, coconut, olive, mustard and almond have been used by Indian women as part of their grooming ritual to keep their hair in good condition.

> **KEY NOTE** When the body is subjected to stress and illness, the skin and hair are often affected, resulting in dryness and sometimes loss of hair. With tension, the scalp becomes tight, restricting the flow of nutrients to the hair and restricting hair growth. Using oils on a regular basis can help to encourage healthy, shiny hair, it can slow down hair loss and soften and moisturise the hair.

- **Almond oil** – being high in nutrients, this oil has a warming effect on the body and is useful for stimulating air growth. It also helps to reduce muscular pain and tightness.
- **Coconut oil** – this is a popular oil for Indian head massage as it is very moisturising on the skin and the hair. It also helps to relieve inflammation and can be useful for dry, brittle hair and hair that has become lifeless due to chemical and physical stress.
- **Mustard oil** – this oil is often found in Indian grocery stores and is one of the most popular oils used in North-West India. The smell is pungent and its effects are very warming on the body. Mustard oil is well known for its abilities to break down congestion and swellings in tense muscles and to relieve pain.
- **Olive oil** – this oil has a strong smell and has stimulating properties which increase heat in the body, thereby, helping to reduce swellings and alleviate muscular tightness and pain.
- **Sesame oil** – this is one of the most popular oils used in India and is high in minerals such as iron and phosphorus. This helps to nourish and protect the hair. It is excellent for dry skin and hair. It can also help to reduce swellings and alleviate muscular pain.

PREPARATION FOR INDIAN HEAD MASSAGE

Therapist Preparation

- Ensure the chair height is suitable for you and your client.
- Prepare the oil for the scalp massage, if required.
- Cleanse your hands before the treatment.
- The therapist stands behind the client and sometimes to the side.

Client Preparation

- Check that the client is suitable for treatment by carrying out a consultation.
- Seat the client comfortably in a chair, ensuring that their legs are uncrossed and their feet are placed on the ground.
- Ask the client to remove any obtrusive jewellery such as necklaces, earrings, noserings and to remove glasses.
- Ask the client to brush their hair to remove any residue of hairspray or mousse, and to remove face make-up.

AN INDIAN HEAD MASSAGE TREATMENT

An Indian head massage involves massage treatment applied to the upper back, upper arms, neck, scalp and head and, although it focuses on massage to the upper part of the body, its effects represent a de-stressing programme for the whole body. The massage usually takes about half an hour if massaging all the parts mentioned above. However, the massage may be shortened to 15 to 20 minutes if treatment is to be offered in the office or workplace.

Start an Indian head massage treatment by laying your hands lightly at the top of the client's shoulders and asking them to take three deep breaths in order to centre and prepare for treatment (Figure 8.1). The hands are then laid lightly over the top of the head and held there for a few moments. This helps the therapist and the client to prepare for treatment. It calms and stills the mind.

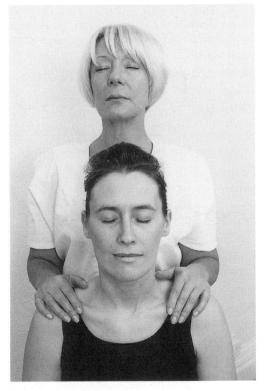

Figure 8.1 Starting position

Upper Back and Shoulders

The shoulders are one of the main areas in which most people hold tension. Indian head massage techniques such as thumb sweeping (Figure 8.2), heel of the hand rubbing (Figure 8.3), and chopping (Figure 8.4) can help to reduce muscular tension across the shoulders and will break down adhesions that may restrict movement.

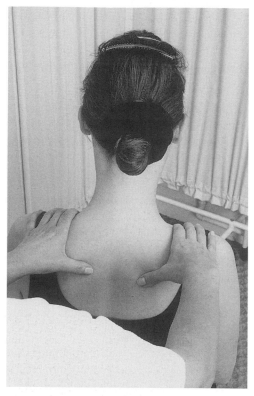

Figure 8.2 Thumb sweeping

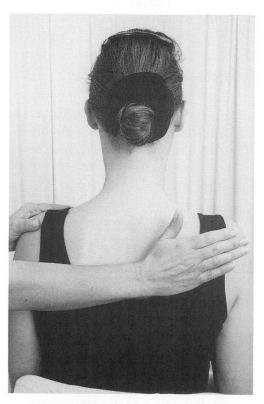

Figure 8.3 Heel of the hand rubbing

Upper Arms Massage

If the shoulders are tense, the upper arms are also likely to be tense. Indian head massage techniques, such as squeezing (Figure 8.5) and smoothing with the forearms (Figure 8.6) can help to increase mobility and flexibility in the arms and shoulders.

Neck Massage

The neck is made up of an elaborate lattice of superficial and deep muscles that are designed to support and move the head and neck. When tense, the neck muscles can cause tension at the back of the skull and lead to headaches and eyestrain. Indian head massage techniques such as thumb pushes to the side of the neck (Figure 8.7) and finger frictions to the base of the skull (Figure 8.8) can help to increase mobility of the neck and reduce tension and tightness.

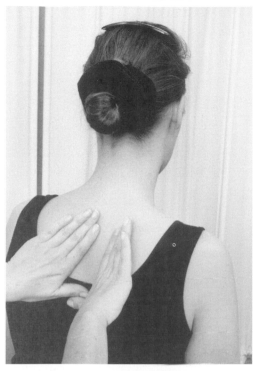

Figure 8.4 Chopping

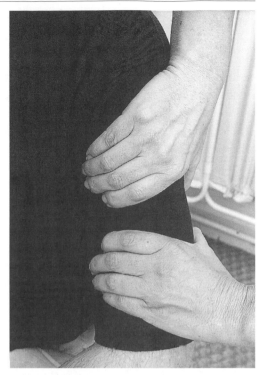

Figure 8.5 Squeezing to the upper arm

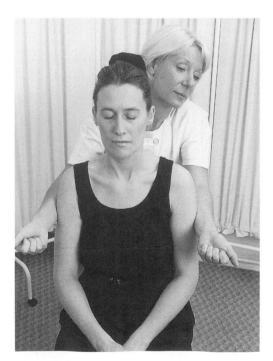

Figure 8.6 Smoothing with the forearms

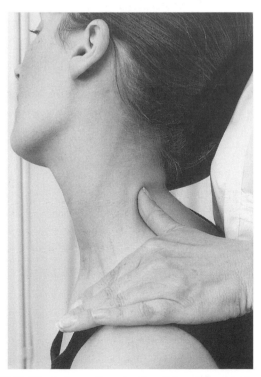

Figure 8.7 Thumb pushes to the side of the neck

Scalp Massage

The scalp has large, broad muscles covering the skull and these tighten with stress, as if creating a tight band across the head. This tension can lead to headaches and neck pain, and can affect the condition of the hair, as the hair roots become constricted and starved of oxygen. Techniques such as whole of the hand frictions (Figure 8.9) and squeezing and lifting on the temples (Figure 8.10) can help to release tightness from the scalp and will stimulate the blood supply to the roots of the hair.

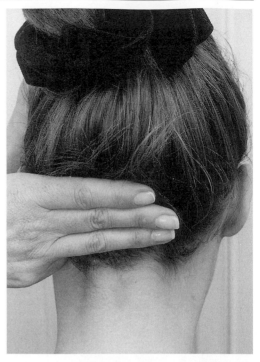

Figure 8.8 Finger frictions to the base of the skull

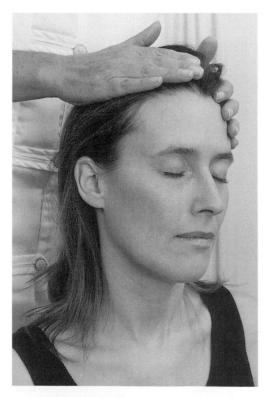

Figure 8.9 Whole hand frictions

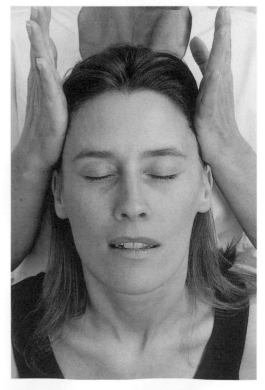

Figure 8.10 Squeezing and lifting on the temples

Face Massage

The face is mainly made up of muscles concerned with facial expression. These are amongst the first muscles to tighten when a person feels stressed and tense. Constant tension in the facial muscles can lead to neck and shoulder problems, as well as headaches and eyestrain.

REACTIONS TO INDIAN HEAD MASSAGE

Indian head massage can cause:

- feelings of tiredness (this is often replaced by a feeling of revitalisation) due to the release of toxins
- relief from stress and muscular tension
- aching and soreness in the muscles, due to the release of toxins and the response of the nerve fibres to the massage
- feelings of calm, peace and tranquillity due to the re-balancing of the chakras
- a heightened emotional state
- feelings of alertness and clear mental thought.

AFTER CARE ADVICE

In order to aid the healing process and to get the maximum benefit from their treatments, clients should be advised to:

- increase their intake of water following treatment to assist the body's detoxification process
- have a suitable rest period after the treatment
- avoid eating a heavy meal after the treatment; try to keep the diet light whilst the body is using its energy for healing
- avoid smoking
- cut down on their consumption of tea, coffee and alcohol
- use oils at home for long-term hair care.

Frequency of Treatment

If part of a stress management programme, Indian head massage should be carried out once or even twice a week for maximum benefit. It is advisable to offer clients a course of treatments (between 4 and 6 initially) and to recommend they take the treatments close together at the beginning.

The frequency of treatment may vary according to a client's time and financial resources. Clients should be encouraged to attend for treatments as often as they can.

CHAPTER 9
Baby massage

INTRODUCTION

Baby massage is an art which encourages loving communication between a parent or carer and their child, through positive physical contact, bonding and stimulation of the child's development. Baby massage has grown in popularity with a greater emphasis being placed on the importance of physical bonding between mother and baby; it is, therefore, not surprising that baby massage instruction classes are becoming a regular feature in GP surgeries and health clinics.

The first few months after having a baby can be a challenging time for parents. Massage can play a vital role in enriching the lives of both the baby and his or her parents by bringing a sense of fulfilment, contentment and well-being. Learning baby massage instruction is a special way for therapists to extend their massage skills, and can be a very rewarding experience.

BENEFITS OF BABY MASSAGE

For a baby, massage begins in the uterus. The uterine contractions during labour stimulate the baby's autonomic nervous system to start the respiratory system and other internal systems which must function independently of the mother. Following birth, there is a period of great change. A new relationship is formed and the demands of the new-born baby become a reality. Bonding with a new-born is not always a natural consequence of motherhood. Massage can help both parents and carers to develop a deeper understanding of the importance of touch. Baby massage can have profound benefits to the baby and its parents. By taking the time to massage their child, parents are helping to teach important qualities such as love, respect and caring.

> **KEY NOTE** Babies, whether premature, underweight or full-term, can benefit from massage. In fact, medical research has shown that massaging premature babies produces better weight gain and increased growth and development.

Benefits for Babies

Massage of a baby by a parent or carer can:
- stimulate the baby's circulation
- stimulate and strengthen the baby's immune system
- soothe and comfort, helping to relieve anxiety and trauma
- promote relaxation and help induce sleep
- aid digestion and elimination (can help relieve colic and constipation)
- encourage muscular co-ordination and joint mobility
- encourage faster weight gain (underweight babies can benefit from an increase in appetite)
- promote fuller and deeper respiration, increasing cell regeneration for growth and development
- improve the appearance and texture of the skin (massaging a baby's skin with oil helps to nourish the skin)
- improve sensory awareness
- enhance neurological and motor development
- promote emotional security and a healthy body image
- stimulation of the skin through massage increases the production of endorphins. This helps to reduce pain and tension, and improves emotional well being by elevating the mood.

Benefits for Parents

Carrying out baby massage has positive effects on the parent or carer too. Massage can:
- deepen and strengthen the relationship between a baby and his or her parents by encouraging bonding
- develop parental confidence for handling their baby
- foster feelings of comfort, trust, enjoyment and security
- help reduce stress in both baby parents, helping them to cope more easily
- provide a period of mutual pleasure for both baby and parents/carer
- help parents to become more aware and understanding of their baby's needs, as the massage becomes a form of loving communication.

THE GROWTH AND DEVELOPMENT OF A BABY FROM BIRTH TO 18 MONTHS

Neonate (new-born baby)

New-born babies maintain the fetal position (curled up with their arms and legs turned inwards towards the body) and gradually extend the arms and legs. The neonate has a range of primitive reflexes such as rooting, sucking and grasping. These survival reflexes are present during the first months of life and after this they are replaced by voluntary actions. The neonate is dependent upon the carer for all his or her physical needs. The only means of communication is by crying. All babies enjoy being cuddled and physical contact with their parents helps to increase their security. Neonates are usually very drowsy for the first few days and gradually become more alert and awake for longer periods.

> **KEY NOTE** It is usual to massage a baby after the first month and once an ample amount of weight has been gained. The GP should approve it. However, new-born babies enjoy having their head and back stroked lightly and this is a nice way for parents or carers to start massaging their baby.

Baby at 1 month

A baby at 1 month maintains a degree of flexion. Their limbs begin to extend with large jerky movements, with the arms more active than the legs. Hands are normally closed but, when open, will grasp a finger if the palm is touched. A 1-month-old baby will continue to sleep for long periods in between feeds and will be wakeful for varying lengths of time. Crying is still the main form of communication, although the baby starts to make throaty noises of pleasure when being spoken to.

At 1 month a baby will:
- smile and respond to voices
- turn the head and eyes towards a light source (the pupils react to light)
- follow a moving object with the eyes.

> **KEY NOTE** The sensory experience of gentle massage and stroking at this stage can help a baby to feel secure and to develop their sense of touch. Care should be taken to support the head at all times due to head lag (the head will fall backwards).

Baby at 3 months

By 3 months, most babies are developing voluntary movements to replace their primitive reflexes. They are wakeful for longer periods of time and show awareness of familiar situations (feeding, bathing) by smiling, cooing and excited limb movements. They are usually alert and will move their head to gaze around.

At 3 months a baby can:
- bring their hands together
- kick vigorously
- hold their head erect for a few seconds
- watch movements of hands and play with fingers
- hold an object briefly but is unable to co-ordinate hands and eyes.

Baby at 6 months

Babies at 6 months are generally lively and sociable. They usually respond by laughing, with loud, tuneful vocalisation (babbling with double syllables, for example mama and dada). The head and eyes of a 6-month-old baby move in all directions. Babies recognise voices and show annoyance.

Physical skills are quite extensive and include:
- sitting with support
- turning the head from side to side
- kicking strongly
- rolling over from front to back
- raising the head
- lifting the legs and grasping the feet
- raising the head and shoulders with hands on floor (when in prone position)
- grasping toys, moving them from one hand to another.

Baby at 9 months

At 9 months, most babies are mobile with a desire to explore. They are usually very attentive to sounds, particularly voices. He or she babbles loudly in a long repetitive string of syllables (mam-mam, da-da) and understands words (no, bye bye) and shouts to attract attention.

A 9-month-old baby will be able to distinguish strangers from familiar faces and will cling to a known adult. At 9 months, a baby will imitate hand-clapping and play peek-a-bo. They begin to develop fine motor skills as they start to balance; they demonstrate very active movements of the whole body and limbs and can:
- sit alone unsupported for 15 minutes or more
- lean forwards without losing their balance
- crawl or roll
- pull themselves to a standing position (falling backwards with a bump)
- support themselves by holding onto a firm object
- manipulate objects with a lively interest
- try to feed themselves.

Baby at 12 to 15 months

At 12 to 15 months, babies usually start walking and will sit and stand without support. At this age, babies can demonstrate affection and can understand simple instructions. They will communicate their wishes and needs.

At 12 to 15 months babies can:
- pick things up with precise movements and place objects down with increasing control
- feed themselves
- build a tower of bricks
- clasp hands together in delight and in play
- hold crayon in palmar grasp and scribble backwards and forwards
- throw a ball and try to catch it
- point to a familiar object in the book.

Baby at 18 months

At 18 months, babies are extremely active, walking and running with arms and legs apart. They will walk upstairs and down with help. They will explore the environment energetically and with increasing understanding.

An 18-month-old baby can use six to 20 words and will attempt to sing. At 18 months, a baby may have bowel and bladder control.

At 18 months babies can:
- pick up small objects on sight using a delicate pincer grasp
- imitate everyday activities
- hand a named object
- take off their socks and shoes
- enjoy putting small objects in and out of containers
- use thumb and fingers to grasp a crayon or pencil and scribble on paper, to-and-fro moments are common and with random dots
- point to a named object.

Stages of Baby Growth and Reaction to Massage

Babies all react differently to massage according to their age and stage of development. During the first 3 months, babies display many neonatal reflexes which may affect their positioning and support whilst being massaged. The moro (startle) reflex may cause the baby to startle when unsupported. Many infants hold their arms in tight with their fists closed and may become anxious when the arms are massaged. It is important for the instructor to advise the carer to be aware of their baby's responses and to encourage stroking in a loving way. They should use a position in which their baby seems happy and most contented. Every baby will be unique in their response and massage should be adjusted upon observation of the baby's behaviour.

After the first 3 months of life, babies start to look around their environment and enjoy reacting with people. They may develop tension in their back due to exercising the muscles in preparation for crawling or walking. They may even roll over during the massage.

Mobility is the major challenge for a baby between 7 and 12 months. They may be so intent on moving that they no longer find massage such a relaxing experience. It is important, therefore, for the instructor to encourage the parent to be inventive with their massage strokes and to make them aware that the baby's tolerance levels will be lower. It may be beneficial to concentrate on massaging specific body parts such as the legs. These may start to hold tension as the baby learns to stand and walk.

For older babies (from the crawling stage onwards), massage techniques are varied to accommodate the growth of the child; it may be possible to apply more pressure depending on the size and the sensitivity of the child and there will be no need for stretching exercises when he or she is mobile.

Working with an older child requires a different approach to massaging an infant. Parents should be advised to try telling stories as they massage to entertain their child's active mind and to alleviate boredom. Using stories will help babies to stimulate all their developing senses.

RELEVANT ANATOMY AND PHYSIOLOGY

The visible changes in the size of a baby as it develops are as a result of changes in bone, muscles and fat.

Bone Development

At birth most of a baby's skeleton is composed of bone. However, some parts, such as the arms, legs, hand and foot bones are made up of cartilage and do not turn into bone (by a process called ossification) until late adolescence. The cartilage continues to grow before ossifying, resulting in the rapid growth which is characteristic of childhood. A new-born baby may have as many as 300 distinct bones, but many of these fuse together as the child grows (the average number of bones in an adult is 206).

At birth, the bones in a baby's skull are not fully ossified and are joined by flexible bands of fibrous tissues called **fontanelles**. This elasticity of the skull enables rapid growth of the brain during the first few years of life. The facial bones on a baby are only very small.

> *KEY NOTE* Babies' bones are softer with a higher water content than adults. Care must be taken to avoid applying too much pressure, which may cause discomfort and injury.

Muscular Development

A baby's muscle fibres are virtually all present at birth. Like their bones, their muscles fibres are initially small and watery, becoming larger and thicker later in childhood. Although a baby can move quite vigorously at birth, their muscles are not fully developed and will grow in length and breadth, and thicken as the baby develops. The most important factors affecting a child's development include the hormones present in the body, physical activity and diet. The more physical activity a baby has, the more strength and co-ordination they will show in their motor development. A new-born baby does not have enough muscle strength or control to support his or her head, but as the muscles start to develop they provide a basis for future development of gross motor skills, such as walking. Massage can be of great benefit in encouraging muscular co-ordination and joint mobility in babies.

> *KEY NOTE* As a baby's muscles make up only a quarter of their total body weight and are underdeveloped initially, it is important to avoid applying too much pressure when massaging. Use mainly the middle and ring fingers to apply the massage strokes in the early stages, before establishing more contact with the palmar surface of the hand as the baby grows in size.

Adipose Tissue

A baby's tissues initially contain a high proportion of fat (known as adipose tissue), which is a protective layer. This subcutaneous fat, which is laid down at approximately 34 weeks prenatally, will eventually disappear as the child develops.

> **KEY NOTE** Although babies have a high proportion of fat which generates heat, they also lose heat very quickly. It is essential that the room in which the massage instruction takes place is maintained at a warm temperature.

THE FETAL CIRCULATION

The fetal circulation differs from that of an adult in that the lungs, digestive organs and kidneys are non-functional, and only begin functioning at birth. The foetus, therefore, receives its oxygen and nutrients by diffusion from the maternal circulation, with metabolic waste products being removed by the maternal circulation.

The foetus is connected to the mother's uterus by a long **umbilical cord** that terminates in the **placenta**. The placenta and the umbilical cord provide the two-way route through which oxygen, nutrients and other materials pass from the mother to the foetus and waste and cellular secretions pass from the foetus to the maternal circulation.

The fetal circulation is, therefore, modified to suit the non-functional respiratory system and the connection with the placenta. Blood passes from the foetus to the placenta via two **umbilical arteries**, which are branches of the **internal iliac arteries** (branches of the aorta). At the placenta waste products are deposited, and oxygen and nutrients are obtained.

The umbilical arteries wind together through the umbilical cord. At the placenta, they divide into many branches that form smaller vessels where exchange takes place. After the exchanges have occurred, the blood rich in oxygen and nutrients emerges from the placenta and is returned to the foetus through a single large **umbilical vein**, which also extends through the umbilical cord. As the umbilical vein enters the foetus it ascends to the level of the liver. The umbilical vein branches upon contact with the fetal liver and most of the blood flows into a vein called the **ductus venosus**, which passes through the liver and joins the fetal inferior vena cava. Placental blood entering the inferior vena cava joins blood from other tissues and is taken into the right atrium of the fetal heart.

Blood entering the fetal right atrium from the superior vena cava is low in oxygen and laden with waste products, while blood from the inferior vena cava is rich in oxygen and nutrients from the placenta. Blood from these two sources mixes in the right atrium. Some of the blood, primarily that from the superior vena cava, flows through the tricuspid valve into the right ventricle. However, some of the blood, mostly blood from the inferior vena cava passes through an opening between the atria called the **foramen ovale**, that diverts blood directly into the left atrium, bypassing the right ventricle. This blood flows into the left ventricle, bypassing the pulmonary circulation and, hence, the lungs.

Blood in the right ventricle is pumped into the pulmonary trunk when the heart contracts. Instead of going to the lungs, however, most of it is diverted to the aorta through a short valve called the **ductus arteriosus**, which shunts blood directly into the aorta at the superior surface of the heart. The ductus arteriosus prevents blood from going into the lungs and sends it directly to the aorta for distribution to the body. The blood in the aorta is carried to all parts of the foetus through the systemic circulation.

> **KEY NOTE** In an adult, venous blood entering the right atrium flows to the right ventricle into the pulmonary trunk. In the fetal heart, much of the blood in the right ventricle is diverted away from the largely non-functional pulmonary circuit, as the fetal respiratory system is not active.
>
> The net effect of the modifications in the fetal circulation is to divert blood away from the non-functioning pulmonary system into the systemic circulation. Functionally, this increases the amount of blood sent through the placenta, thereby increasing the efficiency in the exchange of materials between the foetus and its mother.

Immediately after birth, the following changes occur:
- Blood begins flowing through the pulmonary circulation when the ductus arteriosus contracts by vasoconstriction, atrophies and becomes the **ligamentum arteriosum**.
- In addition to this, the foramen ovale closes to become the **fossa ovalis**, a depression in the interatria septum.
- The right and left atria become completely separated from one another.
- The umbilical vessels undergo degeneration and the digestive and renal arteries and veins begin functioning.

See page 208 for illustration of fetal circulation.

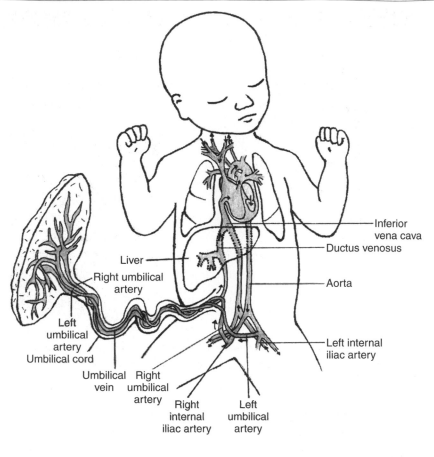

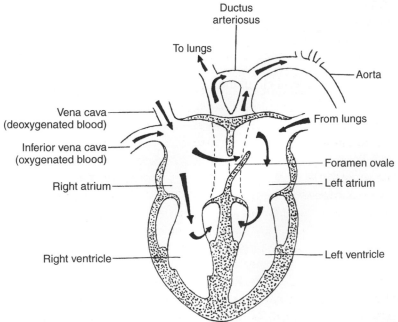

Figure 9.1 The fetal circulation

CAUTIONS AND CONTRA-INDICATIONS FOR BABY MASSAGE

In certain cases it may be necessary to refer the client to their GP before treatment is applied. Where possible, treatment should be adapted to suit the client's condition and needs.

It is essential that, before carrying out a baby massage instruction session, possible contra-indications are discussed with the parents or carers. The parent or carer need to be advised when it may not be possible to massage their baby and why.

Ideally, baby massage should begin after the baby has had their 6 week medical check with their GP, and has received the all clear. However, premature babies may be gently massaged with GP or hospital consent, although the massage may consist of mainly stroking at the initial stages.

The ideal time for massage is when the baby is not too tired or hungry. Advise the parents that the baby should be fed approximately 1 to $1\frac{1}{2}$ hours before the massage session begins. It is also important for the instructor to tell the parents to respect the baby's needs by not massaging when the baby is sleeping or crying.

Parents should seek professional help if their baby is unwell. Parents are invariably the best judges of their baby's health and will realise when the baby does not want to be massaged, but may wish to be comforted and held instead.

> **KEY NOTE** Parents should be encouraged to 'ask' permission from the baby before beginning to massage. They should observe verbal and non-verbal signs from the baby and if he or she is unresponsive to try again at a later stage.

- **Infectious diseases** – parents should be advised that their baby should never be massaged whilst he or she is suffering from an infectious disease to avoid spreading the infection. Babies should never be massaged if suffering from a fever.
- **Recent fractures, sprains and swelling** – parents should be advised to avoid massaging a fracture, sprain or swelling until all signs of inflammation and injury have healed.
- **Recent haemorrhage** – in the case of a recent haemorrhage, massage should be avoided. Parents should be advised to seek medical advice.
- **Recent operation or surgery** – this will depend on the type of surgery undertaken; always encourage the parent to consult the baby's GP or Consultant.
- **Congenital heart condition** – it is essential to take a detailed history of the baby's heart condition, along with the details of any surgical or medical treatment that has been carried out. It is also necessary for the parent to seek clearance from the baby's GP. In general, massage may be helpful due to the relaxation effect, but duration and frequency would need to be decided on an individual basis, depending on the baby's condition and medical advice offered at the time of the proposed treatment.
- **Congenital dislocation of the hip** – in this condition the hip joint is unstable because of a failure to develop properly. It may be associated with the position of the

fetus in the uterus, and there may also be a genetic link. When the hip is dislocated, the head of the femur may become displaced from the socket in the pelvis and, if left untreated, will affect the development of walking. It is important that the baby's hips are tested soon after birth and then at regular intervals up to 1 year. The baby's legs are held in the abducted position by the use of splints. A typical click can be felt as the dislocated head of the femur slips back into its socket.

- **Spastic conditions** – In spastic conditions there is generally an increase in muscle tone which can result in rigidity. Massage may help to increase joint mobility and reduce rigidity, as well as offer comfort and support. Always encourage parents to refer to the baby's GP concerning the nature of the spastic condition.

- **Dysfunction of the nervous system** – this is an umbrella term for disorders of neurological origin. Any dysfunction of the nervous system should be discussed with the GP prior to massage.

- **Epilepsy** – epilepsy is a condition in which there are recurrent attacks of temporary disturbance of brain function. Epilepsy is a complex condition and may take many different forms. The condition will vary with each child and symptoms may range from disturbances in consciousness that are hardly noticeable to mild sensations and lapses of concentration to severe seizures with convulsions. Advise the parent to seek their GP's advice in all cases before proceeding with massage. If massage is advised, keep the sessions brief and monitor the results carefully.

- **Recent immunisation** – it is best to advise parents to wait at least 48 hours to see how the immunisation will affect their baby. (The polio vaccination can, for instance, produce a reaction as it is a live vaccine.) If the baby has no reaction to the vaccination, then the injection site may be treated as a localised contra-indication. After a week, it may be massaged to help disperse any lump that is left.

- **Skin disorders** – a baby's skin is very sensitive and delicate, and any inflammation may be exacerbated by massage. Babies often develop rashes and affected areas should be avoided.

- **Cuts and bruises** – parents should be advised to treat cuts and bruises as localised contra-indications and to avoid the affected area.

Special Care
Premature Babies

It is imperative for parents to seek medical advice before massaging their premature baby. An important consideration is that premature babies' bodies may have been traumatised and areas which may be sensitive include the feet, chest and head. It may be possible for parents to introduce gentle stroking and holding whilst the premature baby is in the neonatal intensive care unit. This can be continued at home to help release the trauma and tension of the hospital environment.

Premature babies may respond to touch and gentle massage most favourably in an area that has been least invaded by equipment (such as the back). Parents can be encouraged to miniaturise each stroke, using a gentle pressure, and to monitor the baby's response.

> **KEY NOTE** It has been proven in practice that premature babies respond positively to gentle stroking and massage. It encourages their growth and development, facilitates the bonding that was lost at the time of birth, and soothes and comforts the baby and its parents/carer.

Conditions and Impairments
Downs Syndrome

This condition is caused by an abnormal chromosome, which affects the child's appearance and development. The condition is usually identified soon after birth by the presence of typical characteristics. Not all children show all characteristics to the same degree, but they have some of the following:

- short hands and feet
- poor muscle tone
- small jaw: tongue appears large
- almond-shaped eyes
- poorly developed nose, sinuses and lungs, with increased susceptibility to infections.

Care should be taken and the parents should be encouraged to consult the baby's GP. However, massage is usually recommended as it helps to increase the tone of muscles and improves balance and co-ordination.

Muscular Dystrophy (Duchenne)

This is a life-threatening condition involving progressive destruction of muscle tissue. The condition only affects boys, as it is an abnormality of the X chromosome, inherited through the female. Advise parents to seek their GP's advice before proceeding with the massage and to exercise caution as muscles will be painful.

The effects of massage can be positive. It may help to slow down muscle atrophy, and lightly massaging over the abdominal area may help with constipation which typically results from the effect of the disorder on the involuntary nervous system.

Spina Bifida

This condition occurs when an area of the spine fails to develop properly before birth. It involves a defect in the fusion of the right and left half of one or more vertebrae during the development of the foetus, resulting in a malformation of the spine. There may or may not be a protrusion of the spinal cord and meninges through the gap.

Advise the parent to seek their GP's advice before proceeding with massage. Massage may help to reduce the spasticity of the muscles and increase joint mobility to help prevent contractures of muscles. However, proceed with extreme caution.

Cerebral Palsy

This is a disorder of movement and posture, in which the part of the brain that controls movement and posture is damaged or fails to develop. Cerebral palsy covers a wide range of impairments in which there may be:

- **Spasticity** – movements are stiff, muscles are tight and limbs are held rigidly and turned in towards the body.
- **Athetosis** – the limbs are floppy and movements are frequent and involuntary.
- **Ataxia** – poor co-ordination and lack of balance.

Advise parents to seek advice from the GP concerning the baby's condition and whether massage is suitable. Generally, massage can be used to help reduce stress, reduce spasticity, prevent contractures, improve posture, improve the circulation to skin and muscles that are used, as well as to provide tremendous emotional support.

Autism

This condition usually occurs from birth. The child has difficulty in relating to other people and making sense of the social world. Advise the parents to seek their GP's advice before proceeding with massage. As autistic children lack an awareness of other people and have problems using non-verbal and verbal communication, any massage given would need to be carefully monitored.

Cystic Fibrosis (CF)

This is a hereditary and life-threatening condition that affects the lungs and the digestive system. It is a recessively inherited condition and, for the child to be affected, both parents must carry the CF gene. It involves breathing difficulties, coughing and repeated chest infections due to the presence of thick and sticky mucus through the airways and into the lungs.

Advise the parent to consult the GP concerning massage for their child. The aim of massage in a child with cystic fibrosis would be to help drain the viscous mucus from the lungs and to increase the blood flow and lymph drainage in the fatigued respiratory muscles. As children with this condition are prone to respiratory infection, it is important to ensure that they do not come into contact with any form of infection.

CONSULTATION AND RECORD KEEPING FOR BABY MASSAGE

A consultation is essential before carrying out the instruction session in order that the instructor may:

- familiarise themselves with the baby and his or her carers
- check whether there are any contra-indications and whether the parent should be advised to seek the GP's advice before massaging
- explain the benefits of baby massage for the baby and its carers
- outline and explain the format of the massage instruction session.

> **KEY NOTE** For ethical reasons it is essential that the parent or guardian consents to the instruction by signing the consultation form and the treatment record.

BABY MASSAGE CONSULTATION FORM

Confidential

Baby's Name: _____ Date of Birth: _____

Parent or Guardian's Name:_____

Address: _____

_____

Tel No:_____ Daytime _____ Evening _____

Has your baby had his/her paediatric check?   Yes ( )   No ( )

Results / Comments: _____

_____

Doctor's Name:_____ Surgery: _____

Health Visitor:_____

Birth details

Type of delivery and weight:_____

Additional information: _____

Weekly weight gain:
above average ( )   average ( )   below average ( )
Sleep pattern:
good ( )   normal ( )   poor ( )
Eating or feeding:
good ( )   normal ( )   poor ( )

Note to Parent or Guardian

The following information is needed for safety reasons before proceeding with the massage instruction. There may be circumstances which mean it may not be possible for you to massage your baby
and you may need to refer to your GP before proceeding.
Do any of the following apply to your baby?

			Dates and Details
Recent operation or surgery	Y ( )	N ( )	_____
Current medical treatment	Y ( )	N ( )	_____
Recent immunisation	Y ( )	N ( )	_____
Skin disorder	Y ( )	N ( )	_____
Recent haemorrhage	Y ( )	N ( )	_____
Recent fracture or sprain	Y ( )	N ( )	_____
Cuts, abrasions or skin rashes	Y ( )	N ( )	_____
Allergies	Y ( )	N ( )	_____
Any dysfunction of the nervous system	Y ( )	N ( )	_____
Spastic condition	Y ( )	N ( )	_____
Any recent or current infections?	Y ( )	N ( )	_____

Are there any other conditions relevant to your baby that have not been mentioned above?

Details _____

Parent or Guardian's Consent

I give my consent to receive baby massage instruction from _____

I understand all information recorded about my baby will be strictly confidential.

Parent or Guardian's signature: _____ Date:_____

RECORD OF BABY MASSAGE INSTRUCTION

Session 1

Date of session: _____   Name of instructor: _____

Type of massage sequence instructed: _____

Oils used: _____

Baby's response to massage: _____

_____

_____

After care advice given: _____

_____

Parent or Guardian's signature: _____

Instructor's signature: _____

Session 2

Feedback from last session: _____

_____

_____

Date of session: _____   Name of instructor: _____

Type of massage sequence instructed: _____

Oils used: _____

Baby's response to massage: _____

_____

_____

After care advice given: _____

_____

Parent or Guardian's signature: _____

Instructor's signature: _____

RECORD OF BABY MASSAGE INSTRUCTION

Session 3

Feedback from last session: _____

_____

_____

Date of session: _____   Name of instructor: _____

Type of massage sequence instructed: _____

Oils used: _____

Baby's response to massage: _____

_____

_____

After care advice given: _____

_____

Parent or Guardian's signature: _____

Instructor's signature: _____

Session 4

Feedback from last session: _____

_____

_____

Date of session: _____   Name of instructor: _____

Type of massage sequence instructed: _____

Oils used: _____

Baby's response to massage: _____

_____

_____

After care advice given: _____

_____

Parent or Guardian's signature: _____

Instructor's signature: _____

PARENTAL FEEDBACK FORM

Please complete this evaluation form to help your Baby Massage Instructor ensure that you have received all the relevant information.

Baby's Name: _____

Parent or Guardian: _____

Instructor: _____

Were all the instructions you received clear, concise and informative?

Yes ( )   No ( )

Comments

Were you given sufficient time to ask questions?

Yes ( )   No ( )

Comments

Did you fully understand how to massage your baby using the relevant massage strokes?

Yes ( )   No ( )

Comments _____

_____

Are there any areas which you are unsure about?

Yes ( )   No ( )

Comments _____

_____

How do you feel about massaging your baby?

_____

_____

_____

Please rate your experience of learning baby massage.

	Low									High
Enjoyable	1	2	3	4	5	6	7	8	9	10
Helpful	1	2	3	4	5	6	7	8	9	10
Interesting	1	2	3	4	5	6	7	8	9	10

Do you have any other comments?

_____

_____

Signed: _____   Parent or Guardian

Date: _____

ETHICS ASSOCIATED WITH BABY MASSAGE PROVISION

As a baby massage instructor, it is important to recognise that babies are aware human beings who deserve respect, tenderness and warmth. Both the baby's and parent's consent should be sought prior to the massage instruction session. The parent may consent by signing the consultation and treatment record. The baby's consent may be offered by the verbal or non-verbal cues given to their carer or to the instructor.

> **KEY NOTE** A code of ethics for Baby Massage Instructors must reflect the fact that a baby has the same rights as an adult, although they are represented by their parent or guardian.

A Code of Ethics for Baby Massage Instruction

- Always carry out a consultation with the parent or guardian to ensure the baby is suitable for massage.
- Always advise the parent or guardian to seek medical advice if the baby is under medical care.
- Ensure that the baby and its parent consent fully to the massage instruction.
- Never abuse the relationship between yourself, the carer and the baby.
- Never give unqualified advice, and use your skills of instruction within the limitations of the therapy and training you have undertaken.
- Ensure that you respect the baby's and the carer's wishes at all times throughout the instruction session, irrespective of their race, creed, colour, sex or religious views.
- Ensure that the working environment provided for the baby massage instruction complies with current health, safety and hygiene legislation.
- Keep accurate, up-to-date and confidential records of treatment and instruction provided.
- Be adequately insured to practice the massage instruction through a professional association.
- Always conduct yourself in a professional manner and be courteous to the baby and carer at all times.

PREPARATION FOR BABY MASSAGE INSTRUCTION

Parents or guardians and the instructor should observe the following hygiene and safety precautions prior to the massage session.

Hygiene precautions for baby massage

1. Always wash your hands before and after commencing the massage.

2. Ensure that you have removed all jewellery which may scratch the baby.
3. Wear comfortable, loose clothing and tie hair back during the massage.
4. Make sure that your nails are short and so that they don't scratch the delicate skin of the baby.

Safety Precautions for Baby Massage

■ Always carry out a thorough consultation with the parent before commencing the session.
■ Refer the parent to their GP if the baby has a medical condition.
■ Do not carry out the massage session if you are suffering from a cold, flu or infectious illness.
■ Prepare a safe environment for the massage session – do not massage in front of an open fire or on a slippery surface.
■ keep hot drinks away from the area.

Preparation for Baby Massage

It is important to advise the parent on how to create the right environment for massage, in order that it is a pleasant and rewarding experience for both parent and child. It is essential that the parent feels relaxed and comfortable before massaging their baby. The following advice should be given to a carer to use as a checklist before massaging:

1. Clear a comfortable space to work in. It should be free from obstructions, wires and unprotected plugs.
2. Ensure that the room is warm and that doors are closed to reduce draughts.
3. Avoid lights which are too bright and glaring.
4. Clear pets from the room.
5. Play some soft music in order to create a relaxing atmosphere.
6. Ensure that you will remain undisturbed for the duration of the massage session.
7. Lay a protective sheet on the floor or table. Cover this with something soft such as a changing mat covered by towels (one large, one medium-sized).
8. Keep plenty of towels at hand in order to keep the baby warm; baby's temperature will drop during the massage. Keep a warm blanket (preferably made from soft cotton) to wrap the baby up in after the massage.
9. Have plenty of tissues or kitchen roll nearby in order to remove any excess oil from your hands. Anti-bacterial wipes are useful.
10. Have a supply of nappies and baby wipes to hand (the relaxation of the massage often makes the baby empty their bladder).
11. Keep oil away from the baby's face.
12. Keep massage oil in a small, leakproof bottle.
13. Have a feeding bottle prepared for your baby for after the massage (cooled, boiled water is recommended).
14. Gently remove baby's clothing, leaving the nappy loose.
15. Wash your hands before starting.

Massage Mediums for Baby Massage

It is very important to advise a parent to select the right medium for baby massage, as a baby's skin is highly sensitive. Cold pressed vegetable oils are best for baby massage as they are full of vitamins and minerals, which will be beneficial for the child's skin. These oils also stay on the surface of the skin for the duration of the massage. Baby oil, which is a mineral oil, is not suitable for baby massage as it does not penetrate the skin. It is designed to prevent moisture entering or leaving the body, by forming a barrier on the surface of the skin.

> **KEY NOTE** If the baby's skin is very sensitive and has a tendency towards allergies, it is important to carry out a patch test before proceeding. This can be done by applying a small amount of oil to the baby's skin and leaving for approximately 30 minutes. An allergic reaction will usually result in red blotches. If the baby is allergic to a particular oil, try an alternative. If the reaction is severe, advise the parent to seek medical advice. Both the instructor and the carer must be aware that nut and wheat-based oils may produce an adverse reaction.

Suitable oils for baby massage include:
- **Almond oil** – this oil is very soothing and calming on a baby's skin. It is suitable for all skin types, but especially for dry and inflamed skins.
- **Calendula** – this is especially suitable for use on babies with very sensitive skins as it has anti-inflammatory and healing properties. It is suitable for all skin types, but especially for the dry and sensitive.
- **Grapeseed oil** – this oil is suitable for all skin types and is a gentle emollient, which can help baby's skin to retain moisture.
- **Olive oil** – this oil is suitable for dry, dehydrated or inflamed skins. It is a good source of vitamin E and is very soothing for baby massage.
- **Sunflower oil** – this oil is suitable for all skin types, especially dry skin. It is excellent for baby massage as it is a light oil and contains high levels of vitamin E.

MASSAGE MOVEMENTS USED IN BABY MASSAGE

Effleurage

This is the main technique used in baby massage. It is a light stroke that maintains the continuity of the massage routine. It soothes, relaxes and increases the circulation and is used as a linking stroke in between other movements. With a very young baby it is often the fingers that initially maintain the contact, rather than the whole palmar surface.

A light touch is all that should be applied for a young baby and a firmer pressure may be used once the baby has increased in size.

Petrissage

This technique involves kneading the soft tissues by lifting, rolling and squeezing them with the fingers and thumbs. This technique helps to release tension in the baby, helps to increase the absorption of nutrients into the tissue and stimulates the elimination of waste.

> **KEY NOTE** It is important that a baby has sufficient tissue density before petrissage is applied.

Frictions

These are circular movements applied with the thumbs or fingers over a small area of the baby's skin. Light pressure is applied on a baby, in contrast to the application of massage in an adult. Frictions help to release tension, increase the circulation locally and aid in the elimination of waste.

Gentle Stretching and Joint Movement

These techniques may also be applied during the baby massage, as they help to increase joint mobility, maintain flexibility of the joints, and increase the development of muscular strength and suppleness.

> **KEY NOTE** It is important, when carrying out gentle stretching or gentle joint movement, that you have the baby's full co-operation and that they are relaxed, otherwise the baby may experience discomfort.

Practical Baby Massage Techniques

Baby massage can be undertaken at home on any comfortable surface, such as a bed, on the floor or on the parent's lap. The most important aspect is that the parent or carer and baby feel relaxed and comfortable in their surroundings. Comfort can be aided by the use of plenty of pillows and supports (particularly if working on a bed) or if working against a hard surface.

The instructor may wish to use a massage plinth in a clinical setting. If so, ensure that there are plenty of supports around the baby and that the instructor and the parent or carer sit at the side or the head of the couch to carry out the massage.

INSTRUCTIONAL TECHNIQUES FOR GROUPS AND INDIVIDUALS

Planning and leaflets

Always prepare an outline plan for an instruction session in order that you can pace the session and keep to the allocated time. It is advisable to prepare an explanatory leaflet that may be given out to the parents prior to or during the introductory session. The pamphlet might include information such as:

■ the benefits and effects of baby massage to baby and parents
■ hygiene and safety precautions
■ times when it may not be safe to massage baby
■ an outline guide to the massage sequence, preferably with illustrations
■ after care advice.

How many sessions?

If you have an individual parent to instruct, you may find that two or three sessions of approximately 1 hour each may be enough to familiarise themselves with the techniques and gain confidence. If instructing a larger group, you may find that you will need four sessions of approximately one hour.

During the first session the instructor becomes familiar with the carer and their baby, and undertakes a consultation. It also gives the carer an opportunity to ask any questions. The instructor should reassure them of any worries or fears they may have before starting.

After the initial consultation, you are ready to start the first session. This will generally involve a demonstration of a 5 minute massage routine, something which can be integrated easily into the busiest of home lives.

During subsequent sessions, the instructor and carer will review the last session and discuss both the baby's response to the massage and how the carer felt. The second session may require a recap of the 5 minute routine, or the carer may feel sufficiently confident to be shown a longer routine.

> **KEY NOTE** Before starting the massage session, it is important to tell the carer that, although you will be demonstrating the techniques as a guide for them to follow, there is no right or wrong way of doing massage. If the baby responds favourably to a particular stroke, then they should be encouraged to repeat it. They should let their instinct and the baby's feedback guide them.

Guidelines for parents and carers

Pointers for parents and carers when massaging their babies:

1. Ensure that you and your baby are comfortable before starting.
2. Maintain contact with your baby at all times during the massage.
3. Try and use a slow, rhythmical pace which will be relaxing for both you and your baby.
4. Maintain eye contact with your baby throughout the massage.
5. Ensure that you feel relaxed before starting.

6. Use a light and soft pressure to start with. Be guided by your instinct and your baby when it comes to increasing the pressure.

7. If your baby becomes distressed during the massage, stop and try again later.

8. Try to relax. Remember that the experience belongs to you and your baby and should be enjoyable for both of you.

Methods of Demonstrating

For the first baby massage instruction session, the techniques may be demonstrated on a baby doll or on a baby. If you are carrying out a one-to-one session, showing the techniques on the baby for the parent to follow may be more useful. If conducting a group session, you will not be able to demonstrate on all the babies and could use dolls for familiarisation. Then do individual demonstrations as you go round the group.

FIVE MINUTE BABY MASSAGE

The objective of the 5 minute massage routine is to familiarise the baby and the carer with gentle touch and massage. Once the carer has learned the techniques, a massage session will only take between 5 and 10 minutes at home. However, when instructing the routine may take as long as 15 to 20 minutes.

> **KEY NOTE** Advise the carer to start by attracting the baby's attention by talking softly and gently. It is important to stress to the parent that their voice will play an important part in their baby's massage. By talking calmly and softly or by singing a lullaby, they will help to create an atmosphere of calm.

Short Routine
To start

1. Apply a small amount of oil to the palm of one hand and rub hands together to warm.

Connecting

2. Perform a long, sweeping, linking effleurage stroke with both hands gently across the chest and shoulders, down the arm and down the trunk to the legs and feet, returning with a superficial stroke. Repeat six times.

Chest

3. Use an X stroke across the chest from one shoulder to the opposite hip using alternate hands. Repeat six times.

4. Perform light circles across the top of the baby's chest muscles with the fingers of both hands. Repeat three times.

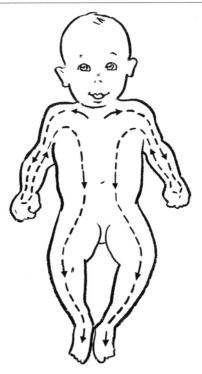

Figure 9.2 Connecting to the front of the body

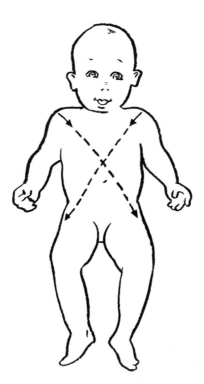

Figure 9.3 X stroke across the chest

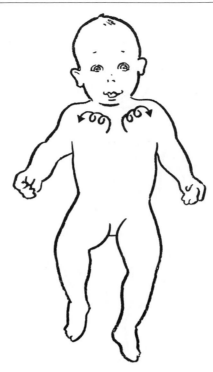

Figure 9.4 Light circles across the top of the chest

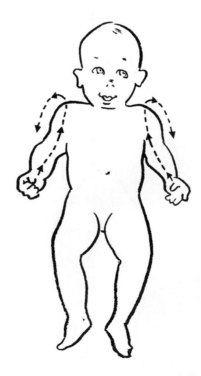

Figure 9.5 Effleurage to the arms

Arms

5. Using alternate hands, apply gently effleurage strokes from the baby's hands up the arm. Circle around the top of arm, returning with a superficial stroke, gently stretching as you glide down. Repeat three times.

6. Perform little circles with the thumbs into the baby's palm.

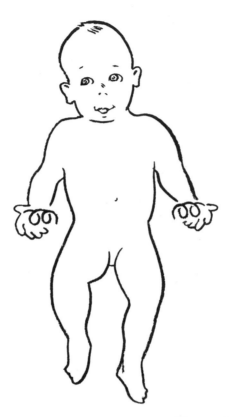

Figure 9.6 Little circles into the palm

Abdomen

7. Make gentle circles around the umbilicus with the tip of the fingers. Repeat three times.

Legs

8. Use gentle effleurage strokes, with alternate hands from the baby's feet, up the legs and around the hips. Return with a superficial stroke, stretching as you glide back down to the toes. Repeat three times.

9. Perform little circles with the thumbs into the sole of the baby's foot. Repeat three times.

Turn baby onto his or her front. The baby may lie on the floor or other surface, or may be placed across the carer's lap.

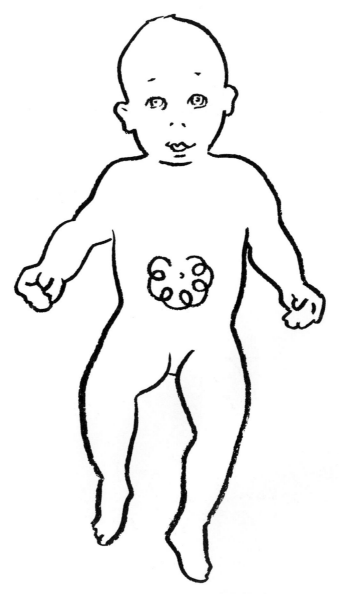

Figure 9.7 Circles around the umbilicus

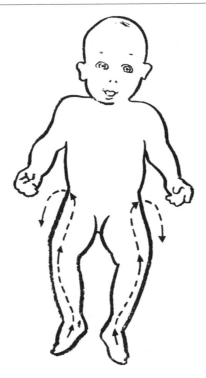

Figure 9.8 Effleurage to the legs

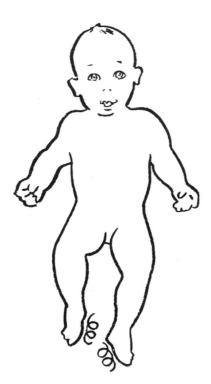

Figure 9.9 Little circles into the soles of the feet

Back

10. Start with a connection stroke using both hands across the baby's shoulders, down the back of the arms, down the back and buttocks to the legs and feet. Repeat six times.
11. Perform the X stroke from shoulder to opposite hip. Repeat six times.

Buttocks

12. Perform broad circles with both hands using the tips of the fingers. Repeat three times.
13. Repeat the connecting stroke down the back of the body (see Figure 9.10). Repeat six times.

Turn baby back onto his or her back.

14. Repeat the connecting stroke down the front of the body (see Figure 9.2). Repeat six times.
15. Finish with gentle leg stretching: make bicycle movements with the legs.

At the end of the massage, advise the parent to wrap their baby up in a towel, give them a kiss, a cuddle and a drink. When ready, remove the oil before dressing.

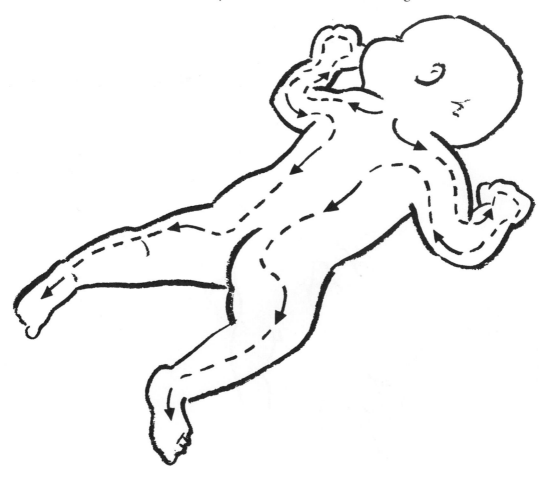

Figure 9.10 Connecting stroke to the back of the body

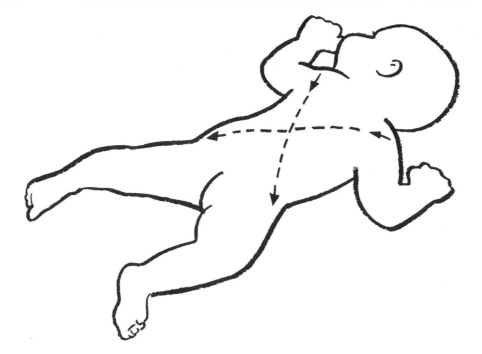

Figure 9.11 X stroke on the back

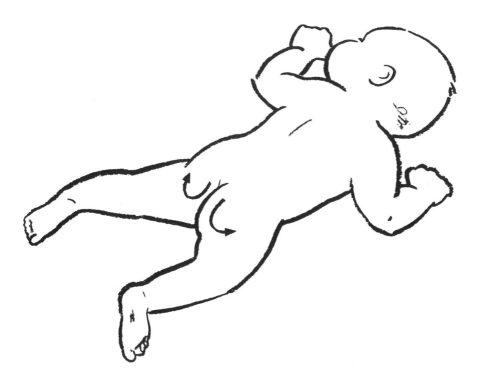

Figure 9.12 Broad circles to the buttocks

LONGER ROUTINE

The longer routine follows a similar pattern to the shorter routine and is a progression from it. Parents should be advised that they may do as much or as little as they feel they can.

Connecting

1. Perform a long, sweeping, linking effleurage stroke with both hands gently across the chest and shoulders, down the arm and down the trunk to the legs and feet, returning with a superficial stroke. Repeat six times.

Chest

2. Use an X stroke across the chest from one shoulder to the opposite hip using alternate hands. Repeat six times.
3. Perform light circles across the top of the baby's chest muscles with the fingers of both hands. Repeat three times.

Front of Arms

4. Using alternate hands, apply gentle effleurage strokes from the baby's hands up the arm. Circle around the top of arm, returning with a superficial stroke, gently stretching as you glide down. Repeat three times.
5. Using one hand with the other to support, gently knead the arm between thumbs and fingers, from the top of the arm down to the hand. Repeat three times.
6. Perform little circles with the thumbs into the baby's palm.

Abdomen

7. Make gentle circles on the solar plexus with the tips of the fingers. Repeat three times.
8. Make gentle circles around the umbilicus with the tip of the fingers. Repeat three times.

Front of legs

9. Use gentle effleurage strokes with alternate hands, from the baby's feet, up the legs and around the hips. Return with a superficial stroke, stretching as you glide back down to the toes. Repeat three times.
10. Using one hand to support, gently knead the legs between the thumb and fingers of the other hand. Travel from the thigh to the foot. Repeat three times.
11. Perform little circles with the thumbs into the sole of the baby's foot. Repeat three times.

Turn baby onto his or her front. The baby may lie on the floor or other surface, or may be placed across the carer's lap.

Back

12. Start with a connection stroke using both hands across the baby's shoulders, down the back of the arms, down the back and buttocks to the legs and feet. Repeat six times.
13. Perform the X stroke from the shoulder to the opposite hip. Repeat six times.
14. Effleurage with both hands up either side of spine and across top of shoulders, returning with a superficial stroke. Repeat six times.
15. Use circular frictions either side of the spine with both hands. Repeat three times.

Back of Arms

16. Using alternate hands, apply gentle effleurage strokes from the baby's hands, up the arm. Circle around the top of arm, returning with a superficial stroke, gently stretching as you glide down. Repeat three times.
17. Using one hand and the other to support, gently knead the arm between thumb and fingers, from the top of arm down to the hand. Repeat three times.

Buttocks

18. Perform broad circles with both hands to both buttocks using the tips of the fingers. Repeat three times.
19. Perform small circular frictions to the one buttock at a time, using the other hand to support. Repeat three times.
20. Use the connecting stroke down the back of the body. Repeat six times.

Back of Legs

21. Use gentle effleurage strokes with alternate hands, from the baby's feet, up the legs and around the hips. Return with a superficial stroke, stretching as you glide back down to the toes. Repeat three times.
22. Using one hand to support, gently knead the legs between the thumb and fingers of the other hand. Move from the thigh to the foot. Repeat three times.

Turn baby back onto his or her back.

23. Use the connecting stroke down the front of the body. Repeat six times.
24. Finish with gentle leg stretching: make bicycle movements with the legs.

If the baby is responsive, you may like to use light circular movements above the temples. Some babies find this a very soothing way to end the massage.

At the end of the massage, advise the carer to wrap their baby up in a towel, give them a kiss, a cuddle and a drink. When ready, remove the oil before dressing.

AFTER CARE ADVICE

Parents and carers should be given after care advice following the massage session. It is particularly useful if the information is available on a handout or leaflet.

Parents and carers should be advised to:
- remove any residue of oil from the skin after the massage and to ensure that all oil is removed before bathing
- avoid exposing the baby to direct sunlight after the massage
- ensure the baby has plenty of fluids after the massage
- allow the baby to sleep or relax after the massage if they want to
- ensure that the baby is kept warm
- monitor the baby's response to the massage
- never leave the baby unattended throughout or after the massage.

FREQUENCY OF BABY MASSAGE

Parents will want to know how often to massage their babies. A baby will benefit most from receiving daily massage for the first six months and, as the child becomes more active, the frequency may be reduced to once or twice a week. However, frequency will be largely dependent on the baby's tolerance and the parent's schedule.

Parents and carers should be encouraged to experiment, massaging at different times of the day to find out what works best for them and their baby. For younger babies, a popular routine is to have a massage followed by a warm bath. The parent/carer and baby can relax together afterwards.

From six months onwards, bath time becomes more of a playtime! At this point, massage generally works better after the bath, when the baby is tired and ready for a nap. Massage before a nap can help baby to sleep more soundly. The most important thing is that the timing of the massage suits the parent/carer and the baby together and that it is a relaxing experience.

CHAPTER 10
Reiki

INTRODUCTION

The word Reiki means 'universal life energy'. It is a natural and simple method of hands-on healing which transfers energy from the giver to the receiver. Reiki energy is a powerful and concentrated form of energy that flows through the hands of a Reiki practitioner. Reiki is a holistic therapy in that it works on the mind, body and spirit by stimulating the body's own natural healing capacity. It is a way of channelling energy positively in order to promote health and to help restore a sense of physical and emotional balance.

Reiki energy is drawn through the channel (the Reiki practitioner) and can only be accessed once the practitioner becomes attuned to it through training with a Reiki Master. Reiki is unique in that the energy is drawn *through* the channel by the recipient, as opposed to being directed by the healer.

Although Reiki is a powerful energy force as a treatment in its own right, many therapists are using Reiki as an additional healing modality to enhance the effectiveness of their other treatments.

Whether you are already a Reiki practitioner or thinking of becoming attuned to Reiki, this chapter will give you a general overview of how Reiki can empower your work as a therapist and how it can become the catalyst for clients seeking a state of balance and harmony.

A BRIEF HISTORY OF REIKI

Reiki is an ancient Japanese form of healing that is thought to date back many thousands of years. Many people believe that the techniques that we use today for healing were first used in India by Buddha and later by Jesus. However, due to the traditional word-of-mouth method of passing knowledge from generation to generation and the lack of documented evidence, we cannot be sure how Reiki originally developed. A great deal of research continues to take place in order to try to establish the original roots of Reiki. We do know that this system of healing, however it was originally conceived, was rediscovered by a Japanese scholar and monk called Mikao Usui. He styled this method of healing and called it Reiki.

Mikao Usui

In the late nineteenth century, Mikao Usui was born into a family that had been practising Zen Buddhism for 11 generations. He was inspired to study the ancient teachings of his ancestors and joined a Zen monastery to begin reading the ancient Sanskrit Sutras. Many years of study led him to references to an ancient form of healing. The texts revealed methods, formulas and symbols that detailed how to practice this art of hands-on healing. However, although Usui had the technical knowledge from his reference material, he lacked the wisdom and deeper insight to enable him to apply this knowledge.

In order to try and find an answer, Usui embarked on a 21-day meditation on a holy mountain near Kyoto. He prayed, fasted, meditated, sang and read the Sutras, asking God to show him the light. On the last day of his fast, he had a remarkable experience whilst meditating. He saw a bright, shining light appear in the sky, which came towards him and struck him in the middle of his forehead (the site of the third eye chakra), leaving him in a state of heightened consciousness. Whilst in this altered state, he recognised the familiar symbols from the Sanskrit Sutras. Simultaneously the application of the symbols and the mantas became clear to him and he became charged with a powerful, healing force.

At the end of his remarkable and enlightening experience, he began his descent from the holy mountain. In his haste, he injured his toe and it began to bleed badly. This led him to his first experience of extraordinary and rapid healing: when he held his hands around his foot, he discovered that the bleeding stopped immediately and the pain had vanished. Usui called his gift from God 'Reiki', Japanese for universal life force.

Usui then spent 7 years helping to heal the beggars in the slums of Kyoto. Through this experience, he learnt that although he had helped to alleviate the physical body of its symptoms of disease, the beggars had not reintegrated themselves into society or taken charge of their own responsibilities. He realised that it was not enough to heal the body physically, but that it was equally important to help heal the spirit and mind.

Usui retreated once again to meditate and this time, was enlightened with the five principles of Reiki:
- Just for today I will not worry.
- Just for today I will not be angry.
- Just for today I will do my work honestly.
- Just for today I will give thanks for my many blessings.
- Just for today I will be kind to my neighbour and every living thing.

By now, Usui had realised how important it was for those who received healing to give something in return; that there should be an exchange of energy between the healer and the recipient. The rest of Usui's life was devoted to promoting the practice and teaching of Reiki healing, through the organisation Usui Shiki Ryoho of Tokyo, which still exists in Japan today.

Usui Sensei (as he was known) died on March 9th 1926 and there is a memorial dedicated to him, the founder of Reiki healing, at the Saihoji Temple in the Suginami district of Tokyo.

Reiki, as styled by Usui, is universal in that it has no dogma or religious beliefs attached to it, so that it can be accepted by any religion or culture.

By the time of his death in 1926, it was thought that Mikao Usui had initiated approximately 19 students to the level of Reiki Master/Teacher, including Dr Chujiro Hayashi who became a well-respected teacher.

Dr Chujiro Hayashi

Dr Chujiro Hayashi, a Japanese physician and retired naval officer, was responsible for training a further 16 Reiki Masters and for creating a structured formula for training. He opened a private Reiki clinic in Tokyo where his students learnt how to apply Reiki and people were treated. Hayashi wrote many reports on the systems he had developed and how they had been used to help treat various ailments and conditions. He also discovered the importance of giving a whole body treatment in order to remove any physical or emotional blocks, and how the universal life energy would go wherever it was needed for healing.

It would seem that Dr Hayashi had developed his own system and had his own set of disciples aside from the Usui Shiki Ryoho. This would explain the proliferation of different methods of Reiki that exist in Japan today.

> **KEY NOTE** From new research, in particular by Frank Arjava Petter, author of the book *Reiki Fire*, it would appear that the organisation which Usui Sensei founded and presided over (Usui Shiki Ryoho) had only five sequential presidents – Mr Ushida, Mr Iichi Taketomi, Mr Yoshiharu Watanabe, Mr Wanami and the present incumbent, Ms Kimiko Koyama.
>
> Therefore, there is a degree of controversy as to the validity of the title 'Grand Master', as stated in the original story. It is stated that the title 'Grand Master' was never part of the Usui Shiki Ryoho of Japan, and consequently it seems that this title was not passed onto Dr Hayashi, as previously believed in the west.

Madam Hawayo Takata

Hawayo Takata, a young Japanese woman living in Hawaii, suffered a number of serious disorders, including a tumour. Whilst in a Japanese hospital awaiting surgery, she was told of the Reiki clinic run by Dr Hayashi. Madam Takata attended the clinic and received regular treatments over a period of four months and, to her surprise, was completely healed. After her remarkable experience at Dr Hayashi's clinic, she decided that she wanted to learn Reiki and set up her own clinic in Hawaii.

She eventually persuaded Dr Hayashi to allow her to work and train at the clinic for 12 months, after which she returned to Hawaii to set up her own Reiki healing practice. In 1938 Dr Hayashi visited Madam Takata and invited her to become the first female Reiki Master.

After Hayashi's death in 1941, Takata continued to teach and heal for many years. It was about this time that the history of Reiki seems to have become distorted, portraying Dr Mikao Usai as a Christian. Madam Takata felt that the American people and those in the Western world held prejudices against the Japanese, and that it would be impossible to promote a method of healing with its roots in Buddhism and Japanese culture.

By the time she had died in 1980, Madame Takata had initiated 22 Reiki Masters, among them her granddaughter Phyllis Lei Furumoto, and Dr Barbara Weber. The partnership between Phyllis Lei Furumoto and Dr Barbara Weber lasted for about a year, after which they split up and continued to work separately.

The Reiki Alliance was formed by Phyllis Lei Furumoto, while Dr Weber formed another association called the American International Reiki Association. Through the Reiki teachers Furumoto and Weber initiated, the system of Reiki healing became known in the Western world.

Many claims have been made about the 'ownership' of the original Reiki. However, whatever label or title is given to it, Reiki is a pure energy. It can not be owned by anyone, and there is no right or wrong way to apply it. As we have seen, Reiki was styled by Usui to be 'universal'.

Today, through the lineage of the Usui method of Reiki, the traditional Reiki system still exists. However, there are many variations that have spread throughout the Western world. Language and cultural barriers have restricted the communication pathways between the original Usui Reiki organisation and the Western world. However, it now seems that the leadership for Reiki lies in Japan where it was originally founded, and claims to ownership and copyright would therefore seem invalid. The inscription on the Usui memorial states that it was Usui Sensei's wish that Reiki be spread throughout the world and that the main focus of Reiki should be to help others.

> **KEY NOTE** Although the teaching of Reiki may vary in content and application, the common element is the utilisation of universal life energy for the highest good. Therefore, the practice of Reiki, as originally styled by Mikao Usui, is based on intuitive guidance. The flexibility of the Usui system means that it is broad enough to encompass the wide range of methods and techniques used today.

HOW REIKI WORKS

The Reiki practitioner is the channel for conducting Reiki. Through the laying on of hands, the natural healing energy flows from the channel and is directed into the body of the receiver. If a client's energy levels are low and they are suffering from physical and emotional imbalance, it can make them more susceptible to illness.

KEY NOTE By channelling positive energy into the body, a Reiki practitioner can help clients to release negative stress and recharge their energy levels, in order to promote a state of balance.

Reiki can help with a wide range of physical and emotional conditions and can bring balance into a person's life.

Reiki is holistic in that it works on a deep and profound level, healing body, mind and spirit.

BENEFITS AND EFFECTS OF REIKI

Unlike other therapeutic bodywork systems, Reiki healing involves a powerful and concentrated form of energy. This means it is not easy to describe the physiological effects of treatment. However, it is still a profoundly powerful healing tool and its benefits are generally far reaching. Reiki is something which has to be experienced and is often impossible to describe clearly in words.

Reiki can help to:
- induce a state of deep relaxation
- relieve pain (physical and emotional)
- accelerate natural healing
- aid the detoxification process of the body
- calm the mind and body, restoring a feeling of peace
- dissolve energy blockages in the body
- focus the mind, helping to negate confusion and help solve problems
- release tension and negative stress
- rebalance the body's energy
- release emotions
- improve health and well-being
- amplify energy levels.

KEY NOTE It is important to recognise that Reiki affects each person differently. Each person's experience is unique and, although the effects may seem outwardly subtle, profound changes may occur inwardly as the body is encouraged to heal itself. Although Reiki may be used to help others, it may also be used for self-healing and to enhance other aspects of both home and work life.

THE PRACTICE OF REIKI

In order to work with Reiki and become a channel for the universal life force, a practitioner has to become attuned to the Reiki energy through a Reiki Master. Traditionally, Reiki training consists of First Degree, Second Degree and Third (Master) Degree levels.

First Degree Reiki

The First Degree Reiki is the first step in Reiki training, and is usually undertaken over a period of 2 days. During the initiation process, a Reiki Master uses the ancient symbols and mantras that were rediscovered by Dr Usui, in order to connect the student to the universal life energy. The energy enters the body through the top of the head and flows through the upper energy centres, known as the chakras, and continues down the arms, leaving the body by radiating from the hands. Once the student has been connected to the universal life force by a series of four attunements or energy transmissions, the energy will automatically start to flow. They can then begin to channel the healing energy of Reiki to themselves and others. The Master will also teach the hand positions for treating the whole body and will describe how Reiki may help certain conditions. As a result of the attunement to Reiki, students find that their psychic, intuitive and creative abilities become enhanced.

As the Reiki energy begins to flow after attunement, a Reiki practitioner starts a 21-day cleansing and detoxification period. The Reiki attunement has a powerful healing influence on the mind, body and spirit, activating all seven chakras, beginning with the root and ending at the crown, each one taking approximately 24 hours. This cycle happens three times. The detoxification period prepares the practitioner's body for healing, and as a result of this the practitioner may experience the physical and emotional effects of cleansing, as old energy patterns are released.

> **KEY NOTE** Once attuned to the Reiki energy, it is important for the practitioner to apply self-healing. This demonstrates their commitment to Reiki and helps them to become more balanced, in order to help others.

Second Degree Reiki

Second Degree Reiki is for those practitioners who have completed First Degree Reiki and who have sufficient experience, application and knowledge of Reiki. Second Degree is, therefore, the next step towards a deepening commitment to Reiki. After a single attunement by a Reiki Master, a Second Degree Reiki practitioner is taught how to use the sacred Reiki symbols, which open out the full potential of the Reiki energy.

The Second Degree Reiki brings new possibilities to the practitioner in that it:
- helps to increase and amplify Reiki energy, which may be used to help others and for self-healing
- enables the Reiki practitioner to send distant healing.

After the Second Degree attunement, the Reiki practitioner finds that their intuitive abilities and their conscious awareness are enhanced, due to an increase in the vibrational energy of the chakras. There is another 21-day cleansing and detoxification period as negative energies are released and the mind and body restores a state of balance.

Second Degree Reiki practitioners find that there are many ways of incorporating the use of the symbols in their work.

> **KEY NOTE** Due to the fact that the Reiki symbols are considered to be confidential and that there are many different applications, it is not within the scope of this book to illustrate them. Furthermore, without the Second Degree attunement, the symbols are ineffective.

Third Degree (Master)

Master Degree Reiki is for those who feel they wish to devote themselves to Reiki and to make a commitment to practice and teach Reiki, as a way of life. A Reiki Practitioner has to achieve sufficient life experience with Reiki before committing to the Master Degree.

The training programme for each Reiki Master is individually tailored and takes some time to complete. Reiki Masters have to revise their knowledge and clarify their skills in order to be able to teach Reiki to others. A Reiki Master-student receives initiation in the fourth Reiki symbol – the Master symbol – in order to lift their Reiki energy to a higher level. Again, the aim is to help others and for self-development.

CAUTIONS AND CONTRA-INDICATIONS FOR REIKI TREATMENT

> **KEY NOTE** It is important to be aware that, although Reiki treatment can help the natural healing process, it is not a substitute for medical treatment or medication. Any client with a medical condition should, therefore, be referred to their GP before any form of Reiki treatment commences. As Reiki is a form of healing energy, it is not necessarily subject to the same precautions as other forms of therapeutic bodywork.
>
> The following information is intended as a guide and practitioners should be encouraged to seek medical advice if they are unsure of the exact nature of a client's condition.

- **Pacemaker** – it is inadvisable to give a Reiki treatment to a client who has a pacemaker, as the vibrational energy of Reiki may alter the rhythm and mechanism of the pacemaker.
- **Infectious diseases and conditions** – a client with an infectious disease or condition should never be given a Reiki treatment due to the risk of spreading the infection and the risk of cross-infection.
- **Epilepsy** – always refer to the client's GP to find out about the type and nature of epilepsy that the client suffers from. Caution is advised due to the complexity of the condition and the theoretical risk that deep relaxation or over stimulation could provoke a convulsion (although this has never been proven in practice).
- **Diabetes** – a Reiki treatment may have an effect on insulin levels in the blood and close monitoring should be undertaken. Some diabetic clients may have acute compli-

cations such as hypoglycaemia, resulting in dizziness, weakness, pallor, rapid heart beat and excessive sweating. In this case it may be advisable for a Reiki practitioner to refer a client to their GP before treating.

■ **Thrombosis** – there is a theoretical risk that a blood clot may become detached from its site of formation and be carried in the body to another part. Always refer to the client's GP for advice on the client's condition before offering treatment.

■ **Severe circulatory disorders** – always refer to the client's GP to find out about the nature of the condition and its severity. If the client suffers with a stress-related circulatory disorder, Reiki may be beneficial due to its deeply relaxing and stress-reducing effects.

■ **High blood pressure** – due to its deeply relaxing effects, Reiki may help to lower blood pressure. If a client has complications associated with high blood pressure, such as heart disease and kidney failure, refer to the client's GP. Clients with high blood pressure can have hypotension due to their medication. Therefore, they should be encouraged to sit and stand up gradually, to avoid dizziness and falls.

■ **Low blood pressure** – care should be taken to ensure that a client who suffers with low blood pressure to sit and stand up gradually to avoid dizziness and falls.

■ **Infectious diseases and conditions** – a client should never be given a Reiki treatment with an infectious disease or condition due to the risk of spreading the infection and the risk of cross-infection.

■ **Cancer and any other terminal illness** – always liaise with the client's GP and the medical team in the hospital, in order to establish the extent of the disease, before proceeding with Reiki treatment. There are many forms of cancer, each with different symptoms and, therefore, requiring different precautions. Although it has never been proven in practice, there is a theoretical risk of spreading pre-cancerous or cancerous cells.

Conditions Which Require Special Consideration

■ **Pregnancy** – although pregnancy is not an illness, it is wise to avoid treating anyone in the first trimester of the pregnancy. Provided the pregnancy is uncomplicated, great benefits may be gained from Reiki during the later stages of pregnancy.

■ **Babies and children** – Reiki energy can help to intensify the relationship between babies and their parents. It is possible to treat babies and children but, for ethical reasons, it is important to ensure that a parent or guardian is present during the treatment. Treatment for a baby or child would be short and a light pressure would be used.

CONSULTATION FOR A REIKI TREATMENT

Before carrying out a Reiki treatment, it is important to carry out a consultation in order to:
■ ensure the client is suitable for treatment
■ explain the Reiki treatment procedure and how it works
■ explain the benefits of Reiki
■ explain what type of reactions may occur
■ establish the client's treatment objectives
■ answer the client's questions about Reiki and allay any fears.

REIKI CONSULTATION FORM

Confidential

Client note

The following information is required for safety reasons and to benefit your health. Reiki is a natural form of healing. However, there may be times when it is necessary for you to consult your GP before treatment can be offered.

Date of initial consultation: _____

Name: _____

Address: _____

Telephone Number: _____

Date of birth: _____

Doctor's Name: _____

Surgery: _____

Medical history   **Dates and details**

_____

_____

_____

_____

Do any of the following conditions apply to you?

Severe Circulatory Disorder   Y ( )   N ( )

Diabetes   Y ( )   N ( )

Epilepsy   Y ( )   N ( )

Pacemaker   Y ( )   N ( )

High or low blood pressure   Y ( )   N ( )

Cancer or terminal illness   Y ( )   N ( )

Infectious disorder   Y ( )   N ( )

Is it possible you may be pregnant? Y ( )   N ( )

Is there any other information about you and your condition that has not been mentioned above?

Details: _____

_____

Are you taking any medication at the moment?   Y ( )   N ( )

Details: _____

_____

Lifestyle: _____

Occupation: _____

Stress levels: high ( )   average ( )   low ( )

Sleep pattern: good ( )   average ( )   poor ( )

Main presenting problem/s:

_____

_____

Have you had Reiki treatment previously?   Y ( )   N ( )

Details/results

_____

_____

Client Declaration

I declare that the information I have given is true and correct and that I am suitable for Reiki healing. I understand that Reiki is a form of healing and does not substitute for medical advice and/or treatment.

Client's signature: _____   Date: _____

PREPARATION FOR REIKI TREATMENT

The beauty of Reiki is that it can be given anywhere. However, in order to create the right setting for a Reiki healing session, it is best to have a dedicated room or area which is conducive to relaxation. Gentle, relaxing music often helps to create the right ambience for healing.

Before a Reiki treatment commences, it is important to:
- carry out a consultation to establish the client's suitability and their needs
- check the height of your treatment couch and that it is safe to use
- help the client onto the treatment couch
- ensure client comfort by offering pillows as support (under the head, knees, ankles)
- check the temperature of the room is warm
- have a spare blanket ready in case the client feels cold during the treatment
- remove all jewellery (both the practitioner and the client)
- ask the client to remove their shoes and loosen tight clothing
- advise the client to keep their arms and legs uncrossed

Record of Reiki Treatments

Date of treatment:_____

Feedback from last treatment:

_____

_____

Treatment plan:

_____

_____

Results/client response:

_____

_____

After care advice given:

_____

_____

Recommendations for future treatment:

_____

_____

- wash hands before and after treatment
- ensure personal hygiene
- have plenty of tissues handy
- ensure that you feel calm, relaxed and focused to give Reiki effectively.

A GUIDE TO GIVING A REIKI TREATMENT

When carrying out a Reiki treatment, there are several factors to be borne in mind:

- Use a relaxed and gentle pressure when placing the hands in the various positions on the body.
- Use the hand positions only as a guide; the hands will feel where the Reiki energy is needed.
- Hands should be slightly cupped with the fingers firmly closed to concentrate the Reiki energy.
- Reiki will travel to where it is needed the most.
- Some clients may experience extreme cold at the position of the practitioner's hands, whilst the practitioner feels intense heat.

■ Watch for non-verbal communication from the client, such as heavy sighing, yawning or limb movements. This usually indicates a shifting of energy.

KEY NOTE Remember that the hand positions are given only as a guide and form the foundation for working with Reiki energy; practitioners should use their intuition to judge where Reiki is needed most. A practitioner's hands may feel hot, cold, tingly or they may feel the energy pulsing through the hands.

Hand Positions for Reiki Treatment

Before starting, ensure the client is comfortable. Offer the client cushions to place under the head, knees and ankles (if required) and offer a tissue to cover the eyes. It is usual to treat each area for approximately 5 minutes. However, there are many ways to practice Reiki. When it is not possible or practical to give a full treatment of between 60 and 90 minutes, specific areas may be treated with Reiki.

Hand Position 1

■ **Client** – lies supine on the couch.
■ **Reiki Practitioner** – stands or sits at the head of the client.

Cup the hands, keeping the fingers tightly together and gently rest them over the client's eyes (one hand either side of the nose) so that hands cover the forehead and the eyes.

KEY NOTE Do not cover the nose; ensure that the client can breathe easily.

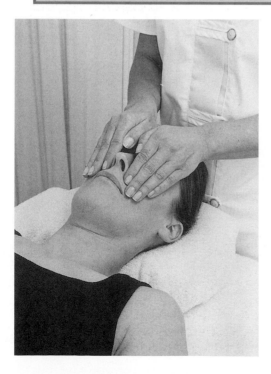

Figure 10.1 Hand position 1

Imbalances that may be helped by Reiki – eye disorders, sinus problems, stress, allergies, headaches, migraine, exhaustion, upper respiratory congestion, hay fever.

Hand Position 2

■ **Practitioner** – sits or stands at the head of the client.

Place your hands on top of the client's head with the palms covering the crown and finger-tips touching the temples, as if you are cupping the head in your hands.

Imbalances that may be helped by Reiki – stress, excessive mental activity, headaches, migraine, head injuries, colds, learning and concentration difficulties.

Hand Position 3

■ **Practitioner** – sits or stands at the head of the client.

Place your hands either side of the client's head and lightly cover the ears.

Imbalances that may be helped by Reiki – problems with balances, hearing and ear problems, tinnitus, colds, flu.

Hand Position 4

■ **Practitioner** – sits or stands at the head of the client

Place your hands at the back of the client's head, covering the occipital ridge.

> **KEY NOTE** Take care with this position and avoid lifting the head or neck. Roll the head to one side to place the first hand at the back of the head. Roll the head gently to the other side to place the other hand.

Imbalances that may be helped by Reiki – headaches, stress, eye problems, sinuses, colds, asthma, hay fever, digestive disorders, depression, fear, shock, head and neck injuries.

Hand Position 5

■ **Practitioner** – sits or stands at the head of the client.

Lightly place your hands over the throat chakra.

> **KEY NOTE** Take care to avoid placing any pressure on the throat if the client has a goitre or feels claustrophobic.

Imbalances that may be helped by Reiki – sore throat, voice and speech problems, problems with self-expression and communication, breathing problems, flu, colds, repressed anger, metabolic disorders.

Hand Position 6

■ **Practitioner** – stands at one side of the couch.

Place both your hands across the upper chest, one either side of the sternum (fingertips of one hand touching the heel of the other hand).

Imbalances that may be helped by Reiki – heart and lung disorders, bronchitis, weakened immunity, general weakness, depression.

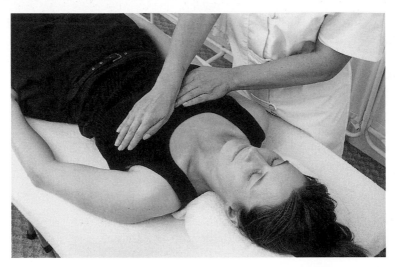

Figure 10.2 Hand position 6

Hand Position 7

■ **Practitioner** – stands at one side of the couch.

Place your hands below the breast, over the lower ribs and above the waist, one hand on each side (fingertips of one hand touching the heel of the other hand).

Imbalances that may be helped by Reiki – digestive problems, immune problems, disorders of the spleen, pancreas or gall bladder, stress (solar plexus) and emotional problems, anger and depression.

Hand Position 8

■ **Practitioner** – stands at one side of the couch.

Place your hands below the waist and across the lower abdominal cavity, one hand on each side (fingertips of one hand touching the heel of the other hand).

Imbalances that may be helped by Reiki – constipation, digestive problems, stress (solar plexus), nausea, indigestion, bloatedness, metabolic disorders, fear, shock and depression.

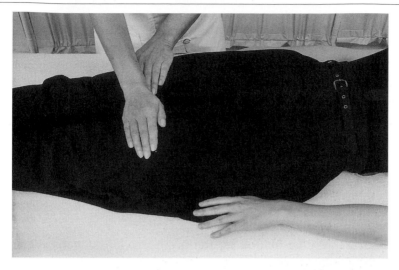

Figure 10.3 Hand position 9

Hand Position 9

■ **Practitioner** – stands at one side of the couch.

Place your hands over the front of the thighs, one hand on each thigh.

Imbalances that may be helped by Reiki – leg and hip injuries.

Hand Position 10

■ **Practitioner** – stands at one side of the couch.

Cup your hands over the knees, one hand on each knee.

Imbalances that may be helped by Reiki – knee joint problems and injuries, fear.

Hand Position 11

■ **Practitioner** – stands at one side of the couch.

Cup your hands over the front of the ankles.

Imbalances that may be helped by Reiki – ankle and foot injuries.

Hand Position 12

■ **Practitioner** – stands at the end of the couch.

Place the palms of your hands over the top of the client's feet (one palm on each foot).

KEY NOTE Holding the hands over the feet helps to balance all the major organs and glands.

Hand Position 13

- ■ **Client** – lies prone.
- ■ **Practitioner** – stands at one side of the couch.

Place your hands across the top of the shoulders, one either side of the spine (fingertips of one hand touching the heel of the other hand).

Imbalances that may be helped by Reiki – neck and shoulder tension, stress, repressed emotions, problems with responsibility.

Hand Position 14

- ■ **Practitioner** – stands at one side of the couch.

Place your hands over the shoulder blades, one either side of the spine (fingertips of one hand touching the heel of the other hand).

Imbalances that may be helped by Reiki – heart and lung disorders, coughs, bronchitis, upper back and shoulder problems, nervousness and tension, depression.

Hand Position 15

- ■ **Practitioner** – stands at one side of the couch.

Place your hands on the lower ribs and above the kidneys, one hand either side of the spine (fingertips of one hand touching the heel of the other hand).

Imbalances that may be helped by Reiki – problems with the kidneys and the adrenal gland, shock, fear, stress, back pain, allergies.

Hand Position 16

- ■ **Practitioner** – stands at one side of the couch.

Place your hands across the lower back, one hand either side of the sacrum (fingertips of one hand touching the heel of the other hand).

Imbalances that may be helped by Reiki – lower back pain, sciatica, hip problems, intestinal disorders, bladder problems, reproductive disorders.

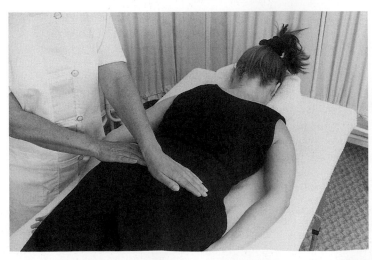

Figure 10.4 Hand position 16

Hand Position 17

■ **Practitioner** – stands at one side of the couch.

Place your hands over the thighs, one hand on each thigh.

Imbalances that may be helped by Reiki – leg and hip injuries.

Hand Position 18

■ **Practitioner** – stands at one side of the couch.

Cup your hands over the back of the knees, one hand on each knee.

Imbalances that may be helped by Reiki – knee joint problems and injuries, fear.

Hand Position 19

■ **Practitioner** – stands at one side of the couch.

Cup hands over the back of the ankles.

Imbalances that may be helped by Reiki – ankle and foot injuries.

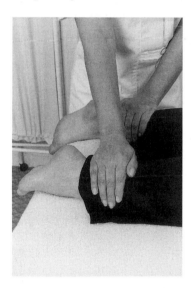

Figure 10.5 Hand position 19

Hand Position 20

■ **Practitioner** – stands at one side of the couch.

Place palms of hands on soles of client's feet (one palm on each foot)

To conclude the treatment

Place your left hand over the client's crown chakra and your right hand at the base of the spine in order to balance the energies. Complete by combing the aura by stroking from the crown down to the feet in a sweeping motion three times.

REACTIONS TO REIKI TREATMENT

Typical reactions to Reiki include:
- sensations of heat or cold
- itchiness
- visualisation of colours
- involuntary movements or twitching
- a pins-and-needles sensation
- emotional responses
- falling asleep
- memory flashes
- sensing the practitioners hands moving.

AFTER REIKI TREATMENT

- Wash or cleanse your hands thoroughly.
- Allow the client to rest for a while after the treatment.
- Help client up from the couch, as they may experience dizziness or drowsiness after treatment.
- Offer the client a glass of water to assist in the detoxification process following treatment.
- Review the client's treatment plan and book their next appointment.

> **KEY NOTE** A client's response to Reiki can be unique and varied. After Reiki, many people report that they either feel deeply relaxed and tired, or energised and refreshed. This may depend on what their body needed at the time of the treatment.

From the information presented in this chapter, it is obvious that there is no definitive guide to practising Reiki. As Reiki is a pure energy, it is not possible to categorise it into right or wrong modes of application. As with all holistic therapies, Reiki can be and should be adapted to suit each client's needs. However it is applied, it should be remembered that Reiki is a simple, natural and powerful form of healing that can help to restore physical and emotional balance.

CHAPTER 11

Stress management

INTRODUCTION

Stress is an unavoidable and inevitable part of modern life. A faster pace of life and ever increasing technological changes mean that we place more and more demands on our bodies. However, despite modern technological changes, the human body is no more able to cope with excessive demands today, than it was in the past. It is now acknowledged that many medical conditions are stress-related and, therefore, more importance is being placed on teaching people to handle stress in order to improve health.

The increase in stress levels is a major factor in the increase in popularity of holistic therapies. The stress relief and relaxation provided by treatments can be beneficial in helping clients to manage their own stress. Holistic therapists need to be aware of stress and how it affects the body, as well as knowing about treatment strategies that may help clients to take control of and manage their own stress.

Stress is something that everyone experiences from time to time and there is no immunity from it. The best way to protect the body from the harmful effects of stress is to learn how to manage it. Mental attitude is a critical factor in dealing with stress, alongside finding ways to reduce the effects of stress. Focusing on the ownership of the sources of the stress, and not on the feelings they generate, is the first step to counterbalancing it.

Stress management can be approached in several different ways. A client's stress management programme will consist typically of a range of holistic therapies, the use of relaxation and stress-reduction techniques, as well as implementing lifestyle changes. Holistic therapists can help clients to recognise their own stress. Therapists can advise on ways to combat stress and can help clients start to manage their own stress positively.

Therapists are not immune to stress. As they are exposed to a considerable amount of emotional energy when dealing with clients,. it is imperative that they learn how to use effective stress management techniques to combat the effects of their own stress.

This chapter gives an overview of stress and stress management, and serves as an introduction to this vast subject. It is beyond the scope of this book to deal with the issue of stress in any greater detail.

DEFINITION OF STRESS

There is no conclusive definition to the word stress. It is a difficult term to define, as stress means different things to different people. However, it can be said that stress is a response to the demands or pressures placed upon individuals. Stress becomes unacceptable when these demands and pressures are noticeable high and beyond the control of the individual.

Stress can be positive in that it can act as a stimulus, increasing levels of alertness. However, it can also be negative when too much stress affects our ability to function effectively.

TYPES OF STRESS

Survival Stress
We experience survival stress when the body reacts to meet the demands of a physically or emotionally threatening situation. The reaction is mediated by the release of the hormone adrenaline, which produces the so-called 'fight or flight' reaction. This type of stress is positive in that it enables the body and mind to react quickly and effectively. When this type of stress occurs over the longer term the on-going release of adrenaline can lead to negative stress.

Internally Generated Stress
This type of stress is often caused by the view or reaction to a situation, rather than the situation itself. Anxiety and worry can lead to negative thought processes and to a feeling that circumstances are out of control. There is a relationship between personality and stress, in particular with anxious and obsessional personalities. Bear in mind that what may be stressful for one person may be enjoyable and exciting for another.

Work or Lifestyle-related Stress
Many stresses that are experienced relate to work or lifestyle. In this context, stress may be generated by some of the following:
- having too much or too little work
- time pressures and deadlines
- the demands of a job with limited resources
- insufficient working or living space
- disorganised working conditions
- limited time, to the detriment of leisure and family life
- pollution
- financial problems
- relationship problems
- ill health
- family situations, such as birth, death, marriage or divorce.

Negative Stress

This type of stress is caused by the inability to manage long-term stress.

HOW TO RECOGNISE STRESS

Recognising stress can be very difficult. It is important to realise that as a person's stress levels increase, their ability to recognise their own stress usually decreases. Stress can manifest itself in different ways, and symptoms may be presented in a number of different ways. These are discussed below.

Short-term Physical Stress Signals

These signals are symptoms of survival stress as the body reacts to situations that are perceived as a threat. Effects of short-term physical stress include an increased heart beat, rapid breathing, increased sweating, tense muscles, a dry mouth, frequency of urination and a feeling of nausea.

Whilst the effects of short-term physical stress may help you to survive in a threatening situation, negative stress may result when the adrenaline is released but a physical reaction is not required. The effects of excess adrenaline can lead to anxiety, frustration, negative thinking, a reduction in self-confidence and distraction. Difficult situations may be seen as a threat rather than a challenge.

Long-term Stress Signals

Common complaints relating to long-term stress are back pain, headaches, aches and pains, excessive tiredness, digestive problems, frequent colds, skin eruptions and exacerbation of asthma. Stress and pressure can also lead to internal and behavioural stress signals.

Internal Stress Signals

When the body is subjected to long-term stress, the mind becomes unable to think clearly and rationally about situations and problems. This can lead to feelings of anxiety, worry, confusion, a sense of being out of control or overwhelmed, restlessness, frustration, irritability, hostility, impatience, helplessness, depression and mood changes. People who suffer from long-term stress may feel more lethargic, have difficulty sleeping, change their eating habits, rely more on medication, drink and smoke more frequently, and have a reduced sex drive.

Behavioural Stress Signals

When people are under pressure, this can be exhibited in some of the following ways: talking too fast, twitching and fiddling, being irritable, defensive, aggressive, irritated, critical and they may overreact emotionally to situations. They may also find that they become more forgetful, make more mistakes, are unable to concentrate, are unrealistic in their judgement and become unreasonably negative in outlook. Pressure may cause some people to neglect their personal appearance and to be increasingly absent from work.

If the body is subjected to excessive short-term stress, it may lead to ineffective performance. This should be treated as a warning sign, and stress management strategies can be adopted to prevent the problem occurring again in the future. The effects of long-term stress, however, can be much more severe. It can lead to extreme fatigue, exhaustion, burn-out and even breakdown.

Summary of the Signs and Symptoms of Stress
Behavioural changes
People who suffer from stress may:

- be argumentative
- be less friendly
- be withdrawn
- avoid friends and relatives
- lose creativeness
- work longer and harder and achieve less
- be reluctant to do their job properly
- procrastinate.

Change of Feelings
People who experience stress may:

- lose their sense of humour
- have a sense of being a failure
- lack self-esteem and have a cynical and bitter attitude
- experience irritability, with conflict at home and work
- feel apathetic.

Change of thinking
Stress can cause people to:

- be rigid in their thinking, with resistance to change
- be suspicious
- have poor concentration
- feel like leaving a job or relationship.

Physical Changes
People may:

- feel tired all the time
- have sleep problems (usually poor sleep)
- be increasingly absent from work, due to prolonged minor illnesses
- have aches and pains
- suffer backache
- experience headaches and migraines
- have indigestion
- hyperventilate
- have palpitations.

Mental Health

The effects of stress can cause feelings of:

■ anxiety
■ depression
■ fear of rejection.

Cognitive Distortion

Stressed individuals may view themselves in a distorted way:

■ **jumping to conclusions** – even in the absence of proof, stressed people may jump to conclusions. They may assume that other people see them in a certain way; they may anticipate that things will turn out badly and act as if their predictions are facts.

■ **all or none** – this is the feeling that, if you fail in one way, you are a total failure. There is a tendency to overgeneralise and to see this single failure as a proof of your life's failure.

■ **mental filter** – this is when people pick out negative events and dwell on them to the exclusion of everything else. Eventually, the positive aspects of life are rejected and ignored.

MANAGING STRESS

Stress management has to take into account each individual's vulnerability to stress. Therapists must be aware of possible sources of stress and be able to identify the signs and symptoms of stress.

> **KEY NOTE** It is very important for therapists to realise that clients are responsible for their own stress and that, very often, it is a by-product of the way they think. When clients come for treatment, therapists do not become in any way responsible for the clients' stress. However, they may contribute in a positive way by suggesting ways in which clients can help to manage their own stress and, thereby, improve the quality of their life.

Therapists are ideally placed to help clients to learn how to manage stress, to help them learn to identify those factors that contribute to it and so be able to control it.

Optimum Stress Levels

Stress levels vary like any other human characteristic. What may seem challenging and exciting to one person, may seem stressful and threatening to another. The most positive approach to successful stress management is to find an optimum stress level which is sufficiently stimulating to allow us to perform well, whilst not becoming overstressed and unhappy.

> **KEY NOTE** It is important for each individual to be able to monitor their own stress levels. Some people operate most effectively at a low level of stress, whilst this may leave another person feeling bored or unmotivated. Alternatively, someone who performs only moderately at a low level, may find they excel at a high level when they are under more pressure.

Stress Diary

The most effective way of finding an optimum level of stress is to keep a stress diary for a short period of time. This provides a method to analyse what is causing the stress and whether it can be controlled effectively. The type of information that can be recorded in a stress diary is the type of stressful event and time, how stressful the event was (on a scale of 1 to 10), what made the event stressful and how the situation was handled. This can provide the key to identifying whether stress was the *cause* or a *symptom* of the event.

When analysing a stress diary, it should be possible to project the following information:
- the level of stress that is optimum for an individual
- the main sources of unpleasant or negative stress
- whether the strategies for managing stress are effective or not.

Managing Stress Effectively

Once there is an understanding or recognition of the causes of the stress and the optimum level for an individual, the next stage is to work out how to manage the stress.

An action plan for managing stress may include:
- ways to control or eliminate the problems that are causing the stress
- using stress-reduction techniques
- making lifestyle changes
- taking a holiday or more frequent breaks
- taking advantage of social and family support
- time management
- making time for hobbies and leisure
- being prepared to ask for help
- looking back at action taken and evaluating the effects.

Stress Reduction

When choosing methods for stress reduction, different strategies may be required for different people and different circumstances.

STRATEGIES FOR COPING WITH STRESS

Planning and anticipating an event or problem that is perceived to be stressful can help to alleviate feelings of stress. Alternatively, it may be the best strategy to avoid an unpleasant and stressful situation, if it is possible to do so. To reduce the perceived importance of a pending, stressful event, plan for it, get it into perspective and reduce the level of uncertainty by seeking as much information as possible.

STRESS-REDUCTION TECHNIQUES

The main objective when managing stress is to help the client to improve the quality of their life and to increase their resistance to stress by employing certain techniques, as well as making lifestyle changes. It is important to realise that, as people react differently to stress, different techniques or combination of techniques may be required for each individual. Stress can only be eliminated if the root causes are recognised and resolved. However, there are ways in which the unpleasant effects of stress may be reduced.

Imagery and Visualisation

Imagery techniques can be useful to create a retreat from stress and pressure, by imagining a place or event that was happy and restful. This image can be called upon over and over again to help manage a stressful period.

Imagery and visualisation are often more effective if imagined pictures are combined with imagined sounds, smell, taste and warmth. For instance, imagining being on a beach, with the warmth of the sun, the water lapping on the shore and the smell of the sea, brings the picture to life. Imagery and visualisation can often be enhanced by a relaxation tape.

Positive Thinking or Cognitive Therapy

Negative thoughts can cause stress, as they can damage confidence and harm effective performance by stifling rational mental thoughts. Common negative thoughts are feelings of inadequacy, self-criticism, dwelling on past mistakes and worrying about how you appear to others. Awareness of negative thoughts can be the first step to counterbalancing stress. It is important to write negative thoughts down and review them rationally. Judge whether they are based on reality. It is useful to counter negative thoughts with positive affirmations, such as 'I can do this', in order to change a negative thought into a positive one.

Meditation

This is a very effective way of relaxing. The idea is to focus your thoughts, leaving the mind and body to recover from the problems and worries that have caused the stress. Meditation can help to reduce stress by slowing down breathing, helping muscular relaxation, reducing blood pressure. It can help clear thinking by focusing and concentrating the mind.

The key to meditation is to quieten the mind and focus completely on one thing. With meditation, it is important for the body to be relaxed and in a comfortable position. Meditation is a very personal experience and can involve a person sitting or lying quietly and focusing the mind. It can be taught in a class situation. Therapists may also facilitate the meditation by using positive mental imagery and visualisation. This helps clients to focus their mind on the imagery and to lift themselves into a state of passive awareness in order to relax.

Breathing

Deep breathing is a very effective method of relaxation and works well combined with other techniques such as relaxation imagery, meditation and progressive muscular relaxation. The experience of any physical or emotional stress will affect breathing. At times of stress, breathing becomes shallow and irregular. The brain can be deprived of oxygen, leading to feelings of dizziness, an inability to concentrate and agitation.

Deep breathing fills the body with positive energy and clears the mind. It can, therefore, prevent stress and can help assert control once feelings of stress have set in.

Breathing Exercise 1

1. Sit or lie in a comfortable position and loosen tight clothing.
2. Place one hand on the chest and the other across the stomach.
3. Inhale deeply through the nose to fill the upper chest cavity and down to the lower part of the lungs, as if breathing into the stomach for a count of 6.
4. Exhale slowly to a count of 12, allowing the air to escape from the top of your lungs first, before the lower part deflates.
5. Repeat this exercise 6 to 8 times.

Breathing Exercise 2

1. Apply the first two fingers of the right hand to the side of the right nostril and press gently to close it.
2. Breathe in slowly through the left nostril and hold for a count of 3.
3. Transfer the first two fingers to the left nostril to close it.
4. Breathe out slowly through the right nostril to a count of 3. Breathe in through the right nostril and hold for a count of 3 and whilst holding transfer the fingers to the right nostril and breathe out.
5. Repeat the exercise 6 times.

Correct breathing is something which really needs to be practised often, until it feels natural. It may then be utilised as a counterbalance to stress. Breathing properly enables the body to relax and regain its natural balance, whilst calming the mind. If a client has difficulty breathing correctly, it may be advisable for them to attend classes which involve structured breathing, such as yoga.

Progressive Muscular Relaxation

This is a physical technique, designed to relax the body when it is tense. It may be applied to any group of muscles in the body, depending on whether one particular area is tense or whether the whole body needs to relax. PMR is achieved by tensing a group of muscles so that they are as tightly contracted as possible. The muscles are held in a state of tension for a few seconds and then relaxed. This should result in a feeling of deep relaxation in the muscles. For maximum effect, this exercise should be combined with breathing exercises and imagery (such as the image of stress leaving the body).

Relaxation Exercise

1. Find a place where you can feel comfortable.
2. Close your eyes and pull your feet towards you as far as you can and hold for a count of 5. Then let them relax. Let them drop as if you are a puppet on a string and the string has broken.
3. Curl your toes as if you are holding a pencil and hold for a count of 5. Then relax.

4. Tighten and tense the calf muscles, count to 5 and then relax.

5. Tighten and tense the thighs, press tightly together, count to 5 and then relax, allowing them to fall apart.

6. Tighten the abdomen, pulling in the muscles, count to 5 and then relax.

7. Tighten the muscles in the hips and the buttocks, count to 5 and then relax.

8. Arch the back and tense the back muscles, count to 5 and then relax.

9. Tense the shoulders by raising them to the ears, count to 5 and then drop them.

10. Lift your arms up with the hands outstretched, as if you are reaching for something. Hold for a slow count of 5 and then let the arms drop down.

11. Tense the muscles in the forehead, count to 5 and then relax.

12. Tense the muscles around the eyes tightly, count to 5 and then relax.

13. Tense the muscles in the jaw and cheeks (as if gritting your teeth), hold for 5 and then relax.

14. By now you should feel relaxed and heavy, as if you are sinking into the floor or chair. Check that all body parts are free from tension. If there are any areas left with tension, hold that part tense again before relaxing. When you're ready, get up gradually, taking your time.

> **KEY NOTE** This exercise is easier to do if the instructions are on tape, preferably spoken by a person with a slow, calm and relaxing voice.

Time Management

Employing time management skills effectively can help to utilise time in the most productive and effective way. Time management can help to reduce stress by facilitating greater productivity and allowing more time to relax. The key factor in time management is to concentrate on *results* and not on *activity* by:

- assessing the value of your time and deciding how it may be used most effectively
- focusing on priorities, deciding which tasks can be delegated and which may be dropped
- managing and avoiding distractions
- finishing work that has been started and working systematically
- learning when to say no and avoid feeling guilty for saying so
- avoiding being someone else's time problem and reduce commitments
- having a planner for the weeks of the years, including a plan for holidays and leisure.

These measures can reduce the effects of long-term stress by helping to put things back into perspective, giving a feeling of control and direction, and freeing up quality time to relax and enjoy life outside of work.

Attitude to Stress

Attitude is a fundamental factor in stress management. A negative attitude can *cause* stress by alienating and irritating other people, whereas a positive attitude can help to draw the positive elements out of a situation, can make life more pleasurable and stress more manageable.

When the body is under stress, it is very easy to lose perspective and relatively minor problems can be perceived as threatening and intimidating.

When faced with a seemingly overwhelming problem it may help to view the problem in a different way, for instance thinking of it as a challenge or concentrating on what may be learned from it, whatever the outcome. It is important to be able to view mistakes as learning experiences and to appreciate that, if something has been learnt from the experience, it has a positive value.

It may help to talk to someone who has had a similar problem. Alternatively, write the problem down in order to put it into perspective. It is also helpful to break the problem down into tasks of a smaller, more manageable size.

Attitude to Other People

Stress can be caused by relationships with other people. Although it is not possible to change a person's personality, a change of attitude may reduce the amount of stress you experienced from your interaction with them. A useful technique to employ when dealing with other people is to try and understand the way they think and why they feel the way they do.

Unfortunately, some people may attempt to exploit a relationship at the expense of the other person. In this case, it is important to project the right approach – by being positive and pleasant but *assertive*. When dealing with a difficult, annoying or frustrating person, it is always a good policy to stay calm (take deep breaths) and neutral in order to be able to think more clearly and react more rationally.

Stress from the Environment

Disorganised living and working conditions can be a major source of stress. A well organised and pleasant environment can make a large contribution to stress reduction and can increase productivity. Stress may be reduced in the environment by improving air quality, lighting, decoration, untidiness and noise levels.

When working in an office, it is advisable to consider the **ergonomics** of furniture as a potential source of stress. If working at a computer station, chairs should be checked for comfort and height. The keyboard and monitor should be positioned properly.

Health and Nutrition

Eating an unbalanced diet can cause stress to the body by depriving it of essential nutrients. Eating a well balanced diet can help to eliminate the chemical stress that may be caused by the consumption of too much caffeine, too much alcohol, high levels of sugar and smoking. Drinking more water may increase energy levels and improve resistance to stress, by clearing toxins from the bloodstream.

Exercise

Taking frequent exercise is one way of reducing stress, as it helps to improve health, relaxes tense muscles, relaxes the mind and helps to induce sleep. Exercise can accelerate the flow of blood through the brain, helping it to function more clearly. It will remove waste products that have built up as a result of intensive mental energy. Exercise also releases chemicals called **endorphins** into the blood stream, giving a feeling of well-being.

When implementing exercise into a stress management programme, consideration should be given to the type of exercise and its suitability for the individual, as if it is difficult or unenjoyable it may *cause* stress. Exercise must be pursued over the long term to derive benefits.

Taking Time Out

A successful way of reducing long-term stress is to take up a hobby with little or no pressure to perform. Long-term stress can also be reduced by taking time out for undirected activities, such as reading a book, taking a walk, having a long bath or listening to music. It is important to take regular holidays or breaks in order to refresh mind and body, and recharge energy levels. Taking a break can also help to put problems into perspective.

Welcoming Change

It is important to realise that, when implementing a stress management programme, there will be an element of change. Success may depend on adapting to the change. Changes in circumstances and lifestyle can be stressful, however it is often the anticipation of the change that is more stressful than the change itself.

Physical and Mental Relaxation

Holistic therapies can help clients to manage their stress. They provide a period of time away from everyday stresses, promote relaxation and allow clients to regain a sense of physical and emotional balance. A combination of relaxation and a holistic therapy programme can relieve tension and stress, and allow the body energies to flow more freely.

Whatever method of therapy is chosen, the key to stress reduction is simply relaxation. When the body reaches a state of relaxation, tense muscles start to unknot, blood pressure starts to lower, breathing becomes more regular and deeper, and the mind drifts into a state of passive awareness.

KEY NOTE Although holistic therapies can provide a positive counterbalance to the negative effects of stress, it is important that a client does not become dependent on a therapist for any advice or service other than the chosen treatment. It is unhealthy for a client to become over reliant on a holistic therapist to deal with their emotional problems or to see them as the one solution to their stress.

The key to successful stress management is for clients to recognise their own stress and for the therapists to guide them as they learn to manage it. Therapists should always remain objective with clients and realise that, by *not* taking responsibility for the clients' problems, they are in fact helping them to help themselves.

CHAPTER 12

Establishing a holistic therapy business

INTRODUCTION

Having the necessary skills and knowledge to practise as a therapist is not sufficient to survive the realities of the business world as a holistic therapist. Acquiring business skills is essential for business success. The purpose of this chapter is to give a general overview of running a successful therapy business. It is beyond the scope of this book to provide a comprehensive business-planning guide; there are many publications and resources listed at the back of this book which are very useful business tools.

Business-planning is an essential part of setting up a business and it encompasses personal beliefs, goals and making and maintaining a professional image. The operation of a business requires many things, including capital (money), motivation, belief in yourself and commitment.

BUSINESS-PLANNING

In order to be successful in your business venture, it is sensible to have a business plan. A business plan will help focus you and your business, and provide direction.

Business plans should be flexible, adaptable and appropriate to the business they relate to. For example, a small business may have a business plan, which is relatively simplistic and can be documented on 3 to 4 sheets of A4 paper, whereas a large company needs a highly detailed business plan, which is usually extensive in length.

Often, small businesses do not have a documented business plan, but rely on information kept in the proprietors' heads. This can be risky, as it is difficult to retain such information and there can be a tendency for the business to just drift along.

With a written business plan, it is much easier to follow a structure, monitor objectives, goals, timescales and follow a strategy to make your business successful, no matter how detailed the plan. A written business plan will also be an essential item, should you ever wish to borrow money from a bank, as they will want to see clearly how your business will function and ultimately 'make money' to repay your loan.

Whatever form your business plan does take, it should exist. Without it, the business is more likely to fail.

You should prepare your own plan as it reflects *your* business and *your* goals. If you are not fully confident or are inexperienced in writing this kind of plan, it is best to seek professional help and guidance. Although the fundamentals of the business plan should come from you, a professional can ensure that the plan is correct, particularly with regard to things such as financial forecasts.

The Contents of the Plan

A typical business plan is structured in a logical format and will usually include the following information (the length and detail of the plan being dependent on the scope of the business venture):

Summary
- an overview of your business and its current status
- brief details of the market, your product and services, your prospective client base and business potential
- objectives and goals, for the short, medium and long term
- summarised financial forecasts for profit
- summarised financial figures of income required

Business Details
- name, address, and contact details
- years trading and legal status, i.e. limited company
- structure, management details, staffing
- SWOT analysis – strengths, weaknesses, opportunities and threats, and how you intend to address them
- goals and objectives, and how they will be achieved
- mission statement and business policies
- products and services

Marketing
- market analysis, size, scope for growth, lifespan
- the market you are targeting

■ the competition you face
■ how you will sell to the market

Business Operational Details
■ location/s of your business
■ operational hours
■ facilities
■ suppliers
■ equipment

Financial Forecasts

This part of the plan must be realistic. In simplistic terms, figures are based on income and expenditure, in order to show profit or loss over a period of time. In other words, your figures will show how much money you have to make in order to pay your expenses and make a profit.

Profit and loss forecasts should be done on a monthly basis, usually shown over a period of three years. This will give a clear, long-term picture.

When detailing your financial forecast, it is essential to include a cash flow analysis and a breakdown of direct and indirect costs. A direct cost is a cost that is associated with providing a single treatment, the cost of the massage oil for example. An indirect cost is a cost that has to be met irrespective of the number of treatments carried out, the cost of rent of the salon for example.

At the end of your plan, it is usual to add appendices. These contain additional information or details relating to previous sections of the business plan.

Review

It is very important to review a business plan at regular intervals to assess progress. If circumstances change it may be necessary to draw up a revised plan.

No two business plans will ever by the same in structure, detail or length. As mentioned previously, this chapter is not intended as a comprehensive or definitive guide. It is, however, designed to highlight the *need* for holistic therapists to have a business plan, and to give you an idea of its purpose and contents.

LEGALITIES OF RUNNING A BUSINESS

Premises

It is advisable to seek legal advice on various aspects of running a business. If leasing or buying premises, you may need to contact the planning department at the local authority, especially if there is a change of use. You will have to undertake the appropriate measures in order to ensure that your business is operating legally.

Employing staff

If employing staff, you are obliged to meet the legal requirements of an employer and, thus, should instigate and observe the relevant laws. Safe and healthy working environments should be maintained as part of your business operations. Your responsibility applies, not just to yourself and your employees, but also to visitors to your premises and members of the public who may be influenced by what you do. When considering the health and safety aspects of your business, fire regulations should be strictly adhered to.

INSURANCE REQUIREMENTS

Essential insurance cover for a holistic therapy business includes:

- **Professional indemnity** – this cover is essential for practising holistic therapists. It provides insurance cover in case you cause injury to a client during a treatment, for example, and the client sues. Most insurance companies offer a minimum of £1 million indemnity cover.
- **Public liability** – this is essential cover and will protect you if a client or member of the public becomes injured whilst on your premises, by slipping on a wet floor for example.
- **Employer's liability** – this is a legal requirement if you employ staff. It protects an employer against any claim brought by an employee who is injured on your premises. A certificate of employer's liability must be displayed on the premises.
- **Product liability** – this type of insurance protects therapists against claims arising from products used. If practising aromatherapy and blending essential oils, it is essential to add a clause to a basic policy covering 'selling-on liability'.
- **Buildings insurance** – this protects buildings against perils such as fire, explosion, flood or storm damage and accidental damage, for example. If working from home, it is important to review your household policy and to tell your insurance company that you will be operating a business from home. If renting, this could be either the landlord's or the tenant's responsibility and should be clarified at the beginning of the tenancy.
- **Contents insurance** – this protects stock, equipment and fittings in your clinic or treatment room against damage or loss. It is important to ensure that you obtain sufficient cover to reflect the replacement value of your contents.
- **Personal accident insurance** – this is an optional insurance policy which protects against loss of income in the event of an accident or illness which prevents you from working. It is important to set aside money for this purpose and to take advice from a professional adviser regarding the best choice of personal accident plan to suit your needs.

RECORD-KEEPING

As with business-planning, record-keeping should be formalised, either in writing or using a computerised format. Records will start to accumulate, whether you want them to or not. Often records grow rapidly and, if they are not documented and organised, they soon become extremely chaotic, even resulting in financial loss. It is, therefore, important to implement a good system for record-keeping, as it will help to ensure that the business runs smoothly. Record-keeping covers financial transactions, records of purchases and records of client treatment for example.

> **KEY NOTE** Accurate record-keeping of treatments is important. Records should be kept up-to-date and should have sufficient detail to ensure continuity of service from one treatment to the next.
>
> If keeping computerised records of clients, it is important to check your responsibilities under the Data Protection Act.

ESTABLISHING YOUR BUSINESS

Staying in business is largely dependent on how clients are treated (will they come back?) and how the treatments are advertised (how do people find out about your business?). It is also dependent on making efficient use of resources, and on your own health.

Success is more likely if you pay attention to the following key aspects of running a business.

Professional Image and Ethics

It is often said that first impressions last, and this applies to the holistic therapy profession. It is important for therapists to project their image in a positive way, by having integrity in their work, by being honest and giving their very best at all times.

A professional image is projected by the personal appearance of the staff, the look of the establishment in which the treatments are provided, the nature of the literature advertising the therapies and how business is systematically and consistently conducted. In order to enhance a business reputation, it is important to identify and play on strengths, but also to make a commitment to strengthen your weaknesses.

Personality

Clients generally prefer to do business with people they like. It is, therefore, important that therapists take time to ensure that clients feel relaxed and comfortable, and that they project a warm and friendly approach.

Telephone Etiquette

It is essential that the business 'phone is answered in a friendly and professional manner. Clients may decide whether to book an appointment, based on how their call is answered. Many therapists have answer machines to monitor their business calls when they are busy with other clients. It is important to ensure that the message is brief and friendly and to return calls promptly.

Developing and Maintaining Good Skills

Whatever type of holistic therapy is practised, it is important to ensure that clients are given the best possible treatment, so that they have a reason to return. It is important for therapists to continue their own professional development by attending courses for advancement. It will help to keep the business alive if they continue to add new dimensions to their work.

Keeping to Treatment Times

Clients are often on a busy schedule and need to be confident that treatment timings will be maintained. For the therapist, there is also the consideration of cost-effectiveness: appointments are charged by time. Bear in mind that, if additional time is allocated to a client's appointment on one occasion, that client will expect that same treatment the next time.

Networking

It is useful for holistic therapists to become acquainted with as many like-minded practitioners as possible: chiropractors, osteopaths, acupuncturists, hypnotherapists, diet and nutrition advisors, for instance. This can help therapists with their professional growth. Practitioners offering different services may also be able to recommend one another to clients.

It is a good idea to ring or write to other professionals, introducing the services that may be offered to their clients and asking to exchange literature that can be given out to clients. Attending local business talks and seminars, or joining the Chamber of Commerce can be a very effective way of networking and of getting known in the local community.

Desire, Determination and Motivation to Succeed

It is important to have all these things in order to succeed in the business world. Without desire, there is no will to succeed. Determination and motivation are attributes which will help a therapist to stay in business. Therapists should not become despondent as most businesses take an average of two years to become established.

Client Comfort and Satisfaction

The way to ensure that a client returns for future treatments is to pay attention to their comfort, and to ensure their needs are being met. Never become complacent with a regular client and always provide a high level of service at all times.

Hygiene and Cleanliness

As holistic therapies involve giving a personal service, clients will be put off by a lack of cleanliness and hygiene, even if the therapist has provided an otherwise good service. Unfortunately, a dissatisfied client will often tell another person, rather than the therapist.

Location of Premises

Consider the location of the therapy centre or treatment room. It is important to address factors such as accessibility, warmth and whether it has a relaxing and comfortable atmosphere. These will all influence whether a client keeps coming for treatments.

It is important to do some research on the neighbourhood and surrounding areas. Clients must feel comfortable and safe as they approach the salon, as well as when they are inside.

WHAT TO EXPECT FROM CLIENTS

Cancellations

It is an unavoidable consequence of working an appointment system that clients cancel. It can be helpful to communicate clearly with all clients if there is a cancellation policy. You may require 24 hours' notice of their cancellation. Some therapists choose to charge a penalty if cancellations are made at short notice. However, this may put some clients off rebooking and, in any case, it is very difficult to enforce.

'No Shows'

From time to time, clients just do not turn up for their appointment. In an attempt to avoid this, some therapists ring to confirm an appointment or to take a deposit if the client is booking a series of treatments. If a client does not have enough respect to ring and cancel, it is best to let the situation go rather than attempting to pursue them.

Complaints

Unfortunately, it is likely that at some point you will get a complaint relating to your business or the service provided. If you're extremely fortunate, you may never receive a complaint. However, it is prudent to be prepared.

Some organisations may have an official complaint procedure in place. Smaller businesses don't usually go to these lengths. However, it is helpful to have an outline procedure to follow in order to deal efficiently with a complaint, with the aim of reaching an agreeable outcome on both sides. Generally, when dealing with a complaint, it is good practice to observe the following guidelines:

- remain calm
- be polite
- listen to the person who is complaining, asking them to explain the nature of their complaint in full
- take the client aside for privacy or, if on the 'phone, try to take the call in private
- do not be aggressive or defensive and do not argue with the client
- do not be passive
- be assertive if appropriate, i.e. if the person complaining is being unreasonable
- assure the person complaining of your best attention
- try and resolve the problem immediately, or as soon as possible.

> **KEY NOTE** Remember that, if complaints are dealt with promptly, in good faith and with excellent customer service, most clients will continue to do business with you. The trouble begins when the client leaves a clinic or puts a phone down *still* feeling dissatisfied. These are the clients who will tell other people.

PRICING SERVICES

One of the most frequently-asked questions by newly-qualified therapists is how much to charge for treatments. Some therapists feel awkward asking for and accepting money for treatments, often failing to realise the value of the service they provide and the value of their skills.

There are several factors to take into consideration when setting prices:

- **Valuing the service provided** – in order for others to value a service, it is important for therapists to value their own work and to view themselves as professionals. It is important to value the time, money and personal sacrifices that are made in order to achieve a qualification and gain experience.
- **Valuing the time spent providing the treatment** – in business 'time is money'. Therefore, it is helpful to consider how much money is required in terms of an hourly rate in order to cover all the overheads and to pay the therapists a good wage. Remember that the therapists' time must be paid for, even when they are not with a client.
- **The expenses involved in providing the treatment** – working out all the expenses involved in providing treatments can be a very good way of setting a realistic price. It is important not to underprice a service, as this indicates that the therapist does not value themselves. People will assume that they are receiving an inferior service if it is too cheap.
- **Local competition** – assess the local competition to give you a good idea of the range of the price scale. Bear in mind that a large establishment may charge higher fees, due to the overheads and staffing levels required. An established and highly experienced therapist may also charge more.
- **Feeling comfortable with the price** – therapists need to feel comfortable with and confident in their fees. They should feel that they offer value for money and that they create an income to suit their needs. If a therapist undervalues their work, they may become resentful and unenthusiastic about their work and it can affect their personal life.
- **Discounts for series bookings** – this can be a useful way of reducing fees to benefit both parties. The client saves money and the therapist gains a regular client, securing payment in advance.
- **Other discount arrangements** – therapists can often benefit from creative marketing opportunities, such as offering a discount to existing clients who introduce a new client, offering a discount off the second treatment provided in a week, or offering a loyalty bonus to regular clients.

PROMOTION OF SERVICES

Marketing is the art of promoting yourself and the services you offer in order to attract clients. There are many marketing strategies that can be used to sell the services you intend to offer. However, one of the most important attributes for a holistic therapist is to have self-confidence, a positive attitude and a belief in their abilities. As the holistic therapy business involves offering a personal service, it is essential that therapists feel confident enough to sell their services and products to potential clients. In order to be able to sell a service or product effectively, it is important for a therapist to:

■ know the services well and have enough experience to be able to sell their benefits to potential clients

■ be aware of the services of competitors, and to have identified their strengths and weaknesses

■ identify with potential clients' needs and to personalise the sale to each individual.

> **KEY NOTE** Some therapists feel uncomfortable with selling. Sales training courses can enhance this very important skill.

METHODS OF SELLING

Selling Face-to-Face

An advantage of this method of selling is that you can project a positive image by the way you look, what you say and the way you say it. Enthusiasm and belief in the product and service, along with a positive and friendly attitude, will often influence clients to book an appointment. Selling face-to-face may be enhanced by attractive leaflets and eye-catching posters which advertise the benefits of treatments.

Selling Over the 'Phone

This type of sale commences from the moment the 'phone is answered. Every call to a salon could be a potential client, so it is important that the 'phone is answered in the most friendly way. When talking on the 'phone, it is important to smile – this helps you to sound friendly.

If clients leave messages on an answerphone, it is essential that these calls are returned promptly and that they are approached in a friendly and welcoming way. Many an initial enquiry can be converted to the sale of an appointment with the right attitude!

By Demonstration or Presentation

This involves presenting or demonstrating the service to a targeted group. A short talk covers the treatment services and benefits and is followed by a demonstration of the techniques. By identifying the target group's needs prior to the presentation, the therapist can personalise the selling.

By Exhibition

Sales exhibitions are an effective way to communicate with lots of potential clients in one place. It is a useful way of distributing brochures and leaflets and of persuading new clients to watch a demonstration or to sample a product or service. When planning an exhibition, it is important to ensure that it is the right type of show for the image of the business and to speak to people who have attended the show before in order to gain feedback from them.

In order to project the right image at an exhibition, it is important to ensure that:

■ the stand is situated to good advantage and is accessible
■ the staff on the stand are approachable and welcoming
■ the stand is attractive, neat and tidy
■ there is space for people to browse without feeling intimidated.

If possible, take the names and contact numbers of those who visit the stand so that you can contact them after the exhibition.

Advertising

Advertising can be a costly business. Therapists should consider the advantages and disadvantages of different types of advertising in order to avoid wasting a limited budget on ineffective methods.

Free Advertising

Some of the most effective forms of advertising are free!

■ **Personal recommendation** – this is the most effective form of advertising for holistic therapies. Potential clients feel more comfortable if they know that they are going to like the person who will provide the service before they book. A certain amount of word-of-mouth advertising occurs naturally as satisfied clients sing the praises of their therapist to other potential clients.

■ **Good public relations** – offering a free talk and demonstration to a particular client group in the community is an ideal way of marketing treatment services, as public interest in holistic therapies is increasing all the time. There are many groups that meet regularly (a list of contact names addresses and phone numbers may be obtained form your local library). If you are going to provide a talk it is important to be prepared and to know as much as possible about the target audience in order that your presentation may be tailored to suit their needs. If you are seen to identify with a particular client group's needs it will create more interest in your treatments. Take a plentiful supply of business cards and promotional literature to hand out at the end of the session.

■ **Publicity in the local paper** – free publicity, which is of interest to local readers, may be available in a free paper. They may be short of news or events that week! For instance, you may be offering a free treatment to those who make a donation to a local charity desperately in need of funds. A story like this would interest your local paper.

When dealing with newspapers, think of a special angle on the publicity, in order to make it out of the ordinary and of interest or value to readers.

Writing a Press Release

A press release is a way of informing journalists of what you are doing, in a format in which they recognise and understand. When writing a press release to send to a newspaper, it is important to consider the following:

■ Relate your information to a current event (such as a charity event) or trend.
■ The press release must be narrowly focussed and highly specific.

- It should be something unusual and something editors don't already know about.
- It should focus on the readers' needs and *not* on the benefits of the service.
- It should educate and be informative.

It is helpful to pick up editorial-style writing by reading magazines and papers. To go with your press release, make up a 'press pack' which includes photographs of topical interest, press cuttings, background information and client testimonials.

Paid-for Advertising

There are several other methods of advertising which may be used in order to reach the potential clients you cannot reach in person, and these include:

- newspaper advertising
- specialist magazines
- national directories
- mailshots
- leaflets and promotional material
- the Internet.

Important considerations when planning an advertisement are:

- Who is your target audience?
- What do you want to say to potential clients?
- How will you communicate to them what you want to say?

Follow the tried-and-tested **AIDA** formula when devising your publicity:

- **A** – attracting **attention** – use an appropriate heading that grabs attention
- **I** – generating **interest** – state what is on offer in an interesting way
- **D** – creating **desire** – say why what you have to offer is needed and desirable
- **A** – motivating **action** – offer the reader an incentive (perhaps a special offer).

Good advertisements are usually targeted to the right audience, accurate and not misleading, catchy, concise and memorable.

> *KEY NOTE* Words that tend to sell in adverts include:
> - you
> - new
> - results
> - health
> - free
> - complimentary
> - benefits
> - now
> - yes!

Local papers

There are two types of advertisements in newspapers and these are **display advertisements\ and business classified**. Display advertising is more expensive and can appear anywhere in the paper, unless you have paid to have a particular space on the front or back page, or on the television page (which can be very expensive), for example.

Display advertising can be a bit of a gamble as it can depend on:
- the day of the week the paper is printed
- the time of the year
- the page the advert appears on
- the layout of the advert in relation to the other advertisers.

An important point to consider with display advertising is that people buy papers for many reasons, not usually to read adverts (the news, announcements and events, crosswords and horoscope all compete for people's attention). So, how is your advert going to grab their attention? Bearing in mind also that newspapers have a short life span.

The person reading the news and features in a paper may come across your display advert but will not be thinking about a massage. They may not be ready to have a massage for some time. In fact, it may take many exposures to your advert before this person feels you are sufficiently familiar to give you a try. It is important, therefore, that adverts are repeated regularly in the same way in order to create a familiarity and that they are memorable. It can help to include a picture of yourself in the advert. This will be eye-catching and will help the potential client to feel they know you.

It is often helpful to give the reader a cause to reply immediately, such as a deadline on a special offer, as this motivates action.

When you have designed an advert, ask friends and colleagues to cast an eye over the design and the wording for critical review. Often a fresh pair of eyes can see things that you have missed.

Display advertising is usually more effective when it is combined with some editorial. Papers often run special features on health-related matters and it may be appropriate to consider a display advert within a feature. The reader is already focused on the subject when they see your advert.

Classified advertising is more cost-effective than display advertising as it is targeted to the service to be provided (adverts are placed together under appropriate headings). The disadvantage with classified advertising is that there may not be an appropriate section for holistic therapies and advertising has to be placed frequently in order to make it effective.

Specialist Magazines

These are usually targeted to a specific audience. Holistic therapists are usually most interested in health-related publications. The main drawback with them are that they are not local, but national. The effectiveness of advertising will depend on the location of the readership and the therapist.

National Directories

Directories such as *Yellow Pages* can be an effective way of advertising. Adverts are targeted by virtue of the fact that entries are classified by therapy type. It is also a long-term form of advertising and can prove to be cost-effective.

Therapists should consider their geographical location and if they are situated between two counties, it may be advisable to take an advert in more than one directory.

Mailshots

These can be a worthwhile exercise, but require a degree of planning and thought. It is better to target a specific group when designing a mailshot, as this will allow you to address the needs of all the potential respondents. Different client groups may need to be approached in different ways.

You could choose to target self-help groups with a common interest in relaxation or you could write to all the Occupational Health Advisors at local companies offering to give free talks and demonstrations as part of their stress management programme. The letter should be sent on headed note paper and be brief and concise. The focus should be on the respondents' needs, although it is helpful to send background information about yourself and your business along with information on the therapies offered.

Mailshots may have a success or response rate of around 2% and this may be enhanced to 5% by follow-up phone calls. Lower response rates are common and a response rate of 10% would be very good indeed.

> **KEY NOTE** If writing to companies, try offering the incentive of corporate membership (a cheaper rate to company employees). This could motivate more clients to use your service. Each employee could be issued with a special card which entitles them to a certain percentage discount.

Leaflets

The content, layout and style of promotional literature, such as leaflets, require careful planning. The AIDA principles are useful and you should consider other factors, such as the colour and general image the leaflet is projecting. It is essential to address the target audience of the leaflet and try to personalise the message for instance: 'Are you feeling stressed and in need of relaxation?' Factors, such as special offers for a limited period, tend to motivate the reader into acting.

Again, ask friends and colleagues to give feedback on how the message comes across and to comment on the design. Think about other leaflets you have seen and try to remember which ones made you respond and why.

Another factor is how the leaflet will be distributed once it has been printed. The most effective form of distribution, albeit time consuming, is to pay a personal visit to target areas in the community. Ask permission for your literature to be displayed. Calling personally will provide you with an opportunity to present a professional image and generate interest. If this is not possible or practical, a well written letter on headed note paper may also be effective, with a follow-up phone call. Prominent places for leaflets to be distributed include health centres, health clinics, GPs' surgeries, schools, universities, community centres, libraries, health clubs and sports centres.

The Internet

Some therapists are now taking advantage of the Internet as a means of advertising their treatments. An attractively designed web page, including a treatment menu and a photograph of the therapist, can promote services to interested parties. Some people feel that the Internet is a little impersonal, but others who are using it regularly feel it is a very efficient means of communication. It is certainly worth considering this as a potential source of enquiries and contact, but remember that not everyone has access to the Internet and that some potential clients may prefer a more traditional means of contact.

FOSTERING REPEAT BUSINESS

The first goal of marketing is to encourage potential clients to try out your services, the second goal is to encourage them to come back again. There is a variety of ways of fostering repeat business:

- create an understanding of the benefits of the treatments you provide to clients and encourage them to book regular treatments
- award loyalty bonuses and implement reward schemes (simple versions of the ones offered by major supermarket chains)
- stay in touch with your clients and inform them of special offers and any new treatments
- invite clients to attend talks and events you may be holding
- always give the best possible service.

STAYING HEALTHY

One of the areas most commonly neglected by therapists, other than acquiring business skills, is their own health and well-being. A therapist can take a number of measures in order to stay healthy whilst working in the holistic therapy profession.

Receive Treatment Regularly

In order to be able to facilitate health and well-being in clients, it is essential that the therapist is in good health. Practising holistic therapies demands a considerable amount of physical and emotional energy. Having regular treatments can help therapists to promote their own overall health and well-being, gaining awareness from the techniques and maintaining credibility with clients.

Body Mechanics

It is very important for therapists to take care with their posture and ensure correct body mechanics in order to avoid stress, strain and injury. Correct body mechanics includes adjusting the height of the couch or chair, keeping the body fit, using body weight effectively, resting the hands in between treating clients, using stretching exercises and using a variety of techniques to avoid sustained pressure.

Exercise

Regular exercise helps to reduce stress and keep the body fit to practice.

Diet

It is important to eat a healthy, well balanced diet and to drink plenty of water in order to have enough energy to carry out the demanding work that practising holistic therapies requires.

Take Time Off

It is important for therapists to take time off for themselves in order to recharge their energy levels.

Resources

ASSOCIATIONS FOR HOLISTIC AND COMPLEMENTARY THERAPIES

Aromatherapy Organisations Council – AOC
PO Box 387
Ipswich IP2 9AN
Members include Professional Aromatherapy Associations and Colleges

The Federation of Holistic Therapists
3rd Floor
Eastleigh House
Upper Market St
Eastleigh
Hants SO50 9FD
The largest organisation in the UK representing beauty, sports and holistic therapists

The Guild of Complementary Practitioners
Liddell House
Liddell Close
Finchampstead
Berkshire RG40 4NS
Represents practitioners of complementary medicine

British Complementary Medicine Association (BCMA)
249 Fosse Road South
Leicester LE3 1AE
The BCMA provides a consultative body for complementary medicine and has its own code of conduct and register of members

Institute for Complementary Medicine (ICM)
PO Box 194
London SW16 1QZ
An independent charity which provides information on complementary medicine to the general public, set up the British Register of Complementary Practitioners in 1989

The Aromatherapy Trade Council
PO Box 52
Market Harborough
Leicestershire LE16 8ZX
The UK authoritative body for the aromatherapy and essential oil trade, members include essential oil suppliers who abide by a strict code of practice regarding marketing, product labelling, bottling and packaging

SUPPLIERS OF HOLISTIC THERAPY GOODS

The Holistic Trading Company
Abacus House
1 Spring Crescent
Portswood
Southampton SO17 2FD
Tel: 02380 363026
Suppliers of high quality essential oils, carriers and bases, posters and training videos

TRAINING

The Holistic Training Centre
Abacus House
1 Spring Crescent
Portswood
Southampton SO17 2FD
Tel: 02380 390982/363026
e-mail: *course information@holistictrainingcentre.co.uk*
Internet address: www.holistictrainingcentre.co.uk
Comprehensive training programme in therapeutic massage therapy, sports massage, remedial massage, aromatherapy, reflexology, Indian head massage, plus a wide range of advanced courses for qualified therapists

JOURNALS

The International Therapist
(Federation of Holistic Therapist members magazine, see page 277)

The Holistic Therapist
1 Granville Walk
Chadderton
Oldham OL9 6SR

The International Journal of Alternative and Complementary Medicine
Green Library
9 Rickett St
Fulham
London SW6 1RU

The Aromatherapist
SPA Ltd
Essentia House
Upper Bond St
Hinckley
Leicestershire LE10 1RS

The International Journal of Aromatherapy
Harcourt Brace & Co Ltd
Robert Stevenson House
1–3 Baxter's Place
Leith Walk
Edinburgh EH1 3AF

Bibliography and further reading

Ashley, Martin, (1999) *Massage – A career at your fingertips*, Enterprise Publishing, ISBN 0 9644662 6 0

Beaver, Marian and Brewster, Jo, (1999) *Babies and Young Children Book 1: Early Years Development*, Stanley Thornes, ISBN 0 7487 3974 2

Beck, Mark F., (1994) *Theory and Practice of Therapeutic Massage*, Milady Publishing Co., ISBN 1 56253 120 4

Byers, Dwight, (1994) *Better Health with Foot Reflexology*, Ingham Publishing Inc., ISBN 0 9611804 2 0

Cohen, Michael H., (1998) *Complementary and Alternative Medicine – Legal Boundaries and Regulatory Perspectives*, The Johns Hopkins University Press, ISBN 0 8018 5689 2

Cox, Gill and Dainow, Sheila, (1988) *Making the Most of Yourself*, Sheldon Press, ISBN 0 85969 478 X

Damian, Peter and Kate, (1995) *Aromatherapy Scent and Psyche*, Healing Arts Press, ISBN 0 89281 530 2

Dougans, Inge, (1998) *Reflexology: A Practical Introduction*, Element Books Ltd., ISBN 1 86204 160 1

Dougans, Inge with Ellis, Suzanne, (1995) *The Art of Reflexology*, Element Books Ltd., ISBN 1 85230 236 4

Falloon, Val, (1992) *How to Get More Clients*, BPCC Wheatons Ltd., ISBN 0 9513347 5 1

Fulder, Stephen, (1997) *The Handbook of Alternative and Complementary Medicine*, Ebury Press, ISBN 0 7493 2665 4

Gardner-Gordon, Joy, (1998) *Pocket Guide to Chakras*, Vibrational Healing Enterprises, ISBN 0 89594 949 0

Hall, Mari, (1997) *Practical Reiki*, Thorsons, ISBN 0 7225 3465 5

Hall, Nicola, (1991) *Reflexology – A Way to Better Health*, Gateway Books, ISBN 0 946551 73 1

Harland, Madeleine and Finn, Glen, (1990) *Healthy Business – The Natural Practitioner's Guide to Success*, Hyden House Ltd., ISBN 1 85623 000 7

Harris, Rhiannon, (1999) *Becoming an Aromatherapist*, How to Books Ltd., ISBN 1 85703 362 0

Honervogt, Tanmaya, (1998) *Reiki – healing and harmony through the hands*, Gaia Books Ltd., ISBN 1 85675 039 6

Lawless, Julia, (1994), *Aromatherapy and the Mind*, Thorsons, ISBN 0 7225 2927 9

Malone, Garry and Adele, (1998) *The Essence of Reiki*, Transceformational Seminars & Publications, ISBN 0 9532620 0 6

Market House Books Ltd., (1998) *Oxford Concise Colour Medical Dictionary*, Oxford University Press, ISBN 0 19 280085 X

McClellan, Sam with Monte, Tom, (1998) *Integrative Acupressure*, The Berkley Publishing Group, ISBN 0 399 52441 X

McClure, Vimala Scheider, (1989) *Infant Massage – A Handbook for Loving Parents*, Bantam Books, ISBN 0 553 34632 6

McGuinness, Helen, (1997) *Aromatherapy – Therapy Basics*, Hodder & Stoughton Educational, ISBN 0 340 67993X

McNamara, Rita J., (1998) *Energetic Bodywork*, Samuel Weiser Inc., ISBN 1 57863 033 9

Pitman, Vicki with MacKenzie, Kay, (1997) *Reflexology – A Practical Approach*, Stanley Thornes, ISBN 0 7487 2867 8

Porter, Anthony J., (1996) *The Practice and Philosophy of Advanced Reflexology Techniques*, ART, ISBN 0 9529066 0 0

Premkumar, Kalyani, (1996) *Pathology A to Z*, VanPub Books, ISBN 0 9680730 0 X

Price, Shirley and Len, (1995), *Aromatherapy for Health Professionals*, Churchill Livingstone, ISBN 0 443 04975 0

Record, Matthew, (1998) *Preparing a Business Plan*, How to Books Ltd., ISBN 1 85703 374 4

Rosser, Mo, (1998) *Body Massage – Therapy Basics*, Hodder & Stoughton Educational, ISBN 0 340 65826 6

Rosser, Mo, (1999) *Body Therapy and Facial Work*, 2nd Edn Hodder & Stoughton Educational, ISBN 0 340 58511 0

Rowlands, Barbara, (1997) *The Which? Guide to Complementary Medicine*, The Penguin Group, ISBN 0 85202 634 X

Salvo, Susan G., (1999) *Massage Therapy – Principles and Practice*, W.B. Saunders Company, ISBN 0 7216 7419 4

Sharamon, Shalila and Baginski, Bodo J., (1997) *The Chakra Handbook*, Lotus Light Publications, ISBN 0 941524 85 X

Stillerman, Elaine, (1992) *Mother Massage*, Dell Publishing, ISBN 0 440 50702 2

Stoppard, Dr Miriam, (1998) *The Baby and Child Health Care Handbook*, Dorling Kindersley, ISBN 0 86318 729 3

Thomson, Hilary and Meggitt, Carolyn, (1997) *Human Growth and Development for Health and Social Care*, Hodder & Stoughton Educational, ISBN 0 340 683627

Walker, Peter, (1995) *Baby Massage – A Practical Guide to Massage and Movement for Babies and Infants*, St Martin's Press, ISBN 0 312 14545 4

Williams, Sara, (1997) *Lloyds Bank Small Business Guide*, Penguin Books, ISBN 0 14 026836 7

Woodham, Anne, (1994) *HEA Guide to Complementary Medicine and Therapies*, Health Education Authority, ISBN 1 85448 903 8

Index

therapeutic massage 103–4
doctors see GP referrals; medical consultation
Down's syndrome, and baby massage 213
drug addicts, and HIV 14
duodenal ulcers 40
DVT (Deep Vein Thrombosis) 36, 38

eczema 17, 26–7
effleurage
    baby massage 219, 224–6
    Indian head massage 192
    therapeutic massage 95–6, 102
Egypt (Ancient) 73, 109
elderly clients
    reflexology 180
    therapeutic massage 104
emphysema 18
endocrine system reflexes 161
endorphins 261
environmental stress 260
epilepsy 27
    aromatherapy 118
    baby massage 210
    Indian head massage 188
    reflexology 166
    Reiki 239
    therapeutic massage 82
ergonomics, and environmental stress 260
erythema 107
essential oils 26, 109, 110–13, 117–44, 146, 147, 150, 153,
    265
establishing a holistic therapy business 262–76
ethics
    baby massage provision 217
    professional 11–12, 266
eucalyptus (Eucalyptus globulus) 131
exercise 260–1, 276

feedback 5, 107
female reproductive system reflexes 164
femoral hernia 30–1
fetal circulation 206
fevers 32, 35, 43, 64, 66
    aromatherapy massage 117, 139
    baby massage 209
    Indian head massage 187, 190
    reflexology 166, 183
    therapeutic massage therapy 82, 93
fibromyalgia 28
fibrosis 102–3
financial forecasts 264
Fitzgerald, Dr William H. 155
foot, anatomy of the 158–9
foot infections, and reflexology 167
fractures
    baby massage 209
    reflexology 165
    therapeutic massage 84
frankincense (Boswellia carteri) 119, 132, 142

frictions 98–9, 102
    baby massage 220
Furumoto, Phyllis Lei 236

Galen 73–4
gall bladder cancer 20
gall bladder meridian 45, 60–2
gall stones 28
gastric ulcers 40
Gattefosse, Dr 110
geranium (Pelargonium graveolens) 132–3, 142
GLC (Gas Liquid Chromatography) 127
gout 16
governing vessel meridians 66
GP referrals 10, 13, 25, 26, 27, 33
    aromatherapy 117–18, 120
    baby massage 209–10, 212
    Indian head massage 187–9
    reflexology 166–7, 174
    Reiki 239–41
    therapeutic massage 82–4, 85
grapeseed oil 145
Greece (Ancient) 73, 109

hacking 100
haemophiliacs 14
haemorrhage
    aromatherapy massage 117
    baby massage 209
    Indian head massage 187, 190
    reflexology 167
    therapeutic massage therapy 82, 87
hay fever 17, 28
Hayashi, Dr Chujiro 235, 236
headaches 2, 28–9, 34–5
health care professionals, liaising with other 9–10
health and nutrition
    stress management 260
    therapists 275–6
heart 2, 82, 83
heart attacks 18, 29
heart chakra 69
heart conditions
    aromatherapy 117
    congenital 24, 209
    Indian head massage 187
    ischaemic 15, 26
    reflexology 166
    Reiki 240
    therapeutic massage therapy 82
heart meridian 44, 46–7
heat–inducing products 95
hepatitis 15, 29–30
hernia 30–1
Herodicus 73
herpes 15
    simplex (cold sores) 31
    zoster (shingles) 31–2
hiatus hernia 30

Guildford College
Learning Resource Centre

Please return on or before the last date shown
This item may be renewed by telephone unless overdue

16/07/05	1 0 DEC 2013	
29/7/05		
1 2 OCT 2005		
– 1 FEB 2006		
– 1 MAR 2006		
– 8 JAN 2007		
– 6 JUN 2011		

Class: 615.822 McG

Title: Holistic Therapies

Author: McGUINNESS Helen